*ten*minute
yoga

Christina Brown

BARNES
& NOBLE
NEW YORK

Contents

This edition published
by Barnes & Noble Publishing, Inc.,
by arrangement with Parragon Publishing.

2004 Barnes & Noble Books

M 10 9 8 7 6 5 4 3 2

ISBN: 0-7607-5027-0

Printed and bound in Indonesia
Produced by the Bridgewater Book Company Ltd.

Introduction

Yoga is not merely a series of exercises simultaneously energizing and relaxing the body, it is a means of harmonizing the mind, body, and spirit and is a great tool of transformation.

In the *Chitta-Vrtti*, a text that codifies the subject, yoga is defined as *chitta-vrtti-nirohdah*, the cessation of the fluctuations of the mind. Yoga is a state of being, not a physical posture.

The aim of yoga is to separate the spirit within from the physical body that acts as its vessel. As the yoga practitioner seeks control over the mind, the thoughts are stilled and the yogi's essential purity is regained. This neutralization of the turnings of thought occurs in a trancelike state known as *samadhi*.

Asana, the use of physical postures, is the practice most commonly equated with yoga in the West. Asana helps to open and prepare the body for the long hours of meditation necessary to reach this goal. It also alters the subtle energies of the body, clearing the path for the experience of higher states.

The word yoga originates from the Sanskrit *yug*, meaning "to yoke." Yoking, or harnessing, energies implies effort, and a goal such as *samadhi* certainly requires discipline. Though the starting point for many people is a few yoga postures, Hatha yoga, sometimes referred to as the "yoga of force," encompasses codes of moral conduct, asanas, breathing practices, concentration, and meditation. These are the tools to achieve union with the cosmic universal power and the state of yoga.

Self-realization and entering samadhi are lofty goals indeed. More realistically, yoga practice has a lot to offer us in the 21st century. By connecting thought, breath, and posture, yoga aligns the mental, physical, and emotional bodies. Yoga practice offers a chance to return to the integrated self and experience the truth of who we are. In experiencing these mini self-realizations we get a glimpse of our essential purity. It is like remembering who we really are, but, caught up in the whirlwind of life, we had forgotten.

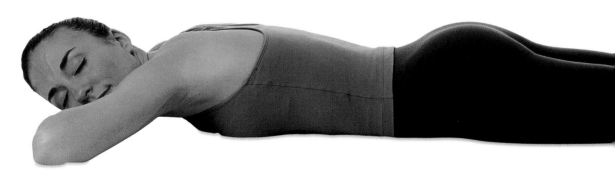

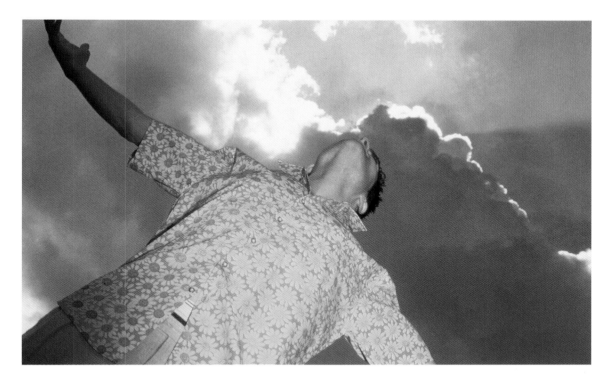

Every yoga practice is a small reversal of consciousness. Yoga teaches us to quieten the mind and observe the present moment. In a refreshing way, our minds are jolted out of our everyday way of thinking. It teaches patience and humbleness in the face of difficulty. We learn to respond to challenges. Yoga expands the heart and gives a sense of wholeness and peace. It is a tremendous tool for transformation.

Ideally yoga should be practiced daily—ten minutes is all it can take for the relaxing powers of yoga to help your mind and body escape from

Yoga will help you to achieve a feeling of unity and wholeness.

the stresses and strains of a busy, modern life. By practicing ten minutes of yoga in the morning and evening, or taking time out from your working day, you can focus your mind and relax your body.

This book contains a selection of postures for you to undertake, and also covers concentration, meditation, and breathing. You should aim to practice a range of different exercises: try pairing one or more asanas in the morning with some meditation or a longer relaxation in the evening. And although these exercises are great for short sessions, when time allows, try an occasional longer session by combining different exercises.

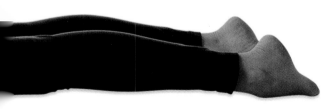

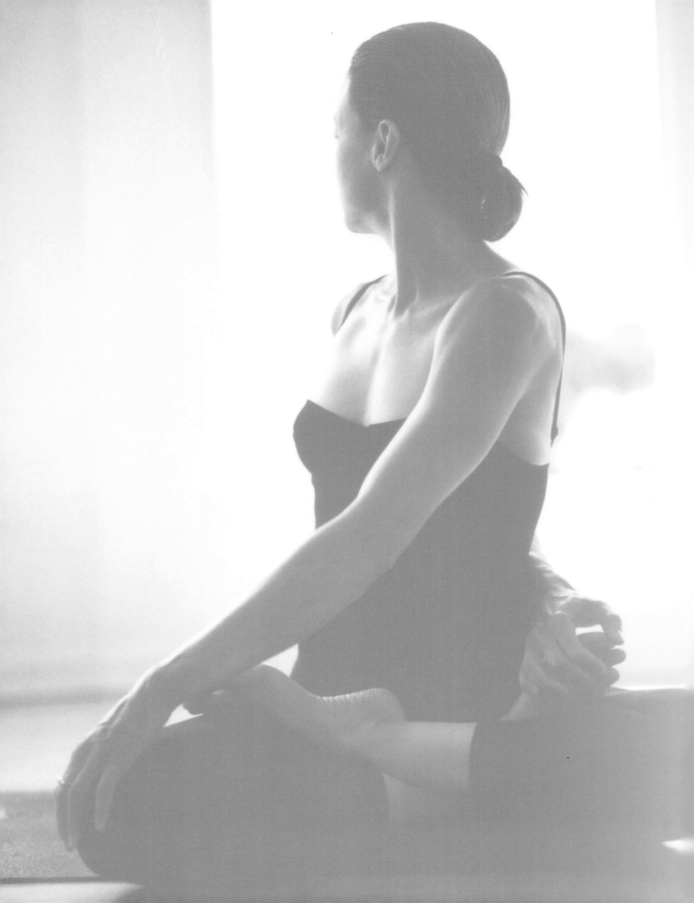

1 BasicsandBackground

After their first yoga class, people often report that they've slept better and feel taller. Yoga has helped people lose weight, overcome fears, conquer habits such as smoking, and develop better concentration, all of which help their performance in their daily tasks. Others feel improved self-awareness, a deeper sense of well-being, developed compassion, enhanced relationships, greater self-acceptance, and a sensation of being at peace.

As we nudge our physical boundaries with yoga postures, we become fully focused on the body.

asana and alignment

Yoga postures are based on ancient geometrical shapes. When performed with attention to alignment, these asanas redesign the body. Muscles are trained to lengthen out of their habitual tense, shortened holding patterns.

Sometimes a tight area of the body is compensating for another weaker area. This area of higher tension can finally lessen this protective holding as the weaker zone strengthens. Even bones can, and do, change shape over time. Bone cells are constantly broken down and new cells laid down where they will best sustain the force of the most common daily impacts. Often we are not fully aware of how we hold and carry ourselves. To help undo less than optimal holding patterns, you should try to attend classes with an experienced teacher who can give you the necessary feedback on your alignment.

Asanas assist the rhythmic pulsations of the body. Blood and cerebrospinal fluid circulation, digestion, excretion, lymphatic drainage, and all the organs in the body require rhythmic pulsation to maintain good health. Yoga postures, by freeing up the body for these natural pulsations, aid good health. Practicing yoga postures is much like giving yourself a massage, not just to the muscles, but to the deeper tissues and internal organs too. In this way, asanas are an excellent form of do-it-yourself preventative medicine.

Asanas work on more than just a physical level. They take the intelligence normally considered to reside in the mind and spread it throughout the entire body. Consciousness can reach everywhere. In the perfect asana, the mind is so engrossed that there is no room for other thoughts to arise. Asanas have psycho-spiritual effects. They influence the emotions and express qualities of the heart.

By aligning the outer body, asanas improve the energy flow in the inner body and help keep, build, and control the vital force, the *prana*.

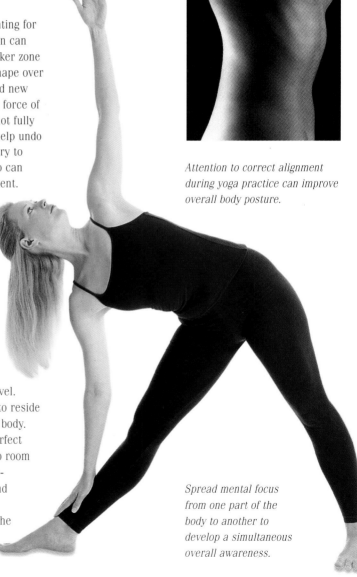

Attention to correct alignment during yoga practice can improve overall body posture.

Spread mental focus from one part of the body to another to develop a simultaneous overall awareness.

One of the most common mental blocks for a beginner is the belief that they are not flexible enough for yoga. However, if you perform a pose with honest effort and correct alignment, you will achieve a result similar to that of someone who seems more flexible. Do not despair about your seeming lack of flexibility; the true measure of your asana is being mentally present—aware of the whole body—and developing your breath.

Breathing

The mind and breath are interrelated; an alteration in one affects the other. By nature, the breath is more constant than the mind. The mind can multiply in ways the breath cannot. Focusing on the breath in asana practice helps to calm the consciousness. For this reason, you should never force the breath. Inhalations and exhalations are like waves breaking on the shore. Keep them even to develop evenness in the mind.

Conscious breathing in a pose will deepen your awareness and keep your mind free of distraction. The breath is your monitor of how you are doing in the pose. When the breath is perfectly steady, your asana is closer to being perfected.

Breathe through the nose, not the mouth, so the air is filtered and warmed. Perform asanas with Ujjayi breathing (see page 113). As a general rule, inhale when you come up out of a pose, when raising the arms, and during movements that expand the chest such as bending backward. Exhale when moving downward, lowering the arms, or bending forward.

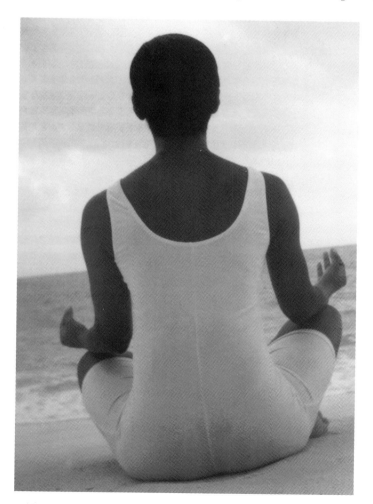

For centuries, yogis have known that calming the breath helps to quieten the mind.

awareness, focus and *being present*

Approach your practice as you can your life. Delight in the small joys.

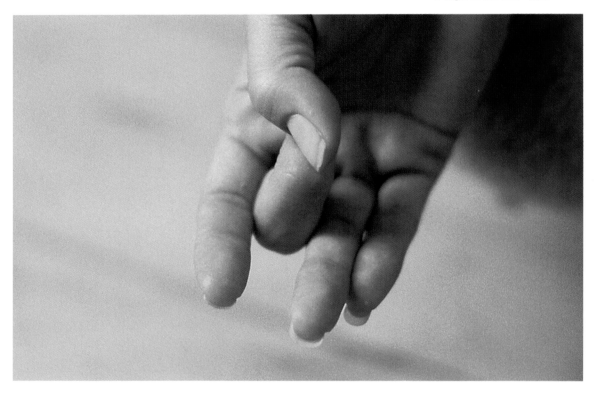

When an asana is performed with full awareness, it develops into something far greater than just a fitness regime. Work with integrity. Become absorbed in the subtle sensations of the body. From observing your hamstring in a forward bend, for example, spread your awareness to the whole leg, then to your lower back without forgetting the original point, radiate your awareness out until it touches the entire body. The essence of yoga is not about twisting yourself into complicated pretzel shapes. Doing the most difficult-looking asanas is not the goal. Rather, mastery of an asana comes when a perfect awareness of the whole body and breath can be maintained.

Working consciously focuses your attention right at the present moment. You may spend one minute in a posture. During this minute, you let go, observe, and refine, seeking the still point, the epicenter of consciousness. During yoga, these minutes link together. If each asana is a pearl, an asana practice forms a beautiful necklace. Over time, this "one minute" focus can extend into your day-to-day life. Yoga is practicing being in the "now." Give attention to the breath, which will bring you back to the present. When you are fully in the present, worries about the future dissipate. Stress floats away when you can release the past and let go of concerns for the future.

Effort

Fully engaging a muscle helps to bring the mind right to that area. Engaging a muscle group increases awareness and is good practice for concentration and being in the now. When the muscles are engaged, the mind is engaged—one reason why asanas have transformative power. The effort required teaches discipline and is rewarding.

For beginners, holding a posture might require 90% effort. It is hard to feel the surrender and release that is the other 10%. With time and dedication, this percentage shifts. The asana becomes more comfortable and feels more rewarding, as the effort it demands falls to 80%, then 70%, and so on. Experiencing the freedom in the pose by yielding into it is sweetly satisfying.

There needs to be a balance between effort and surrender. If you don't extend yourself fully, the practice will be too easy, and your attention will wander. When you overextend yourself, it becomes so difficult that your practice will not be joyful. Practicing with effort doesn't mean using excess force. Frowning, clenching your jaw, or holding your breath are signs to back off. If you feel competitive, try to let go of your over-ambitiousness. Your practice is a metaphor for life. Delight in it.

Surrender

Life experiences build up like layers and are stored in the cellular memory of our bodies. The asanas allow you to explore and soften the unconscious holding on. Yoga helps us to strip off the superfluous emotional overlays that hold us back. There is a sense of freedom and peace within at discovering our true essence.

We are accustomed to the concept of using effort to get somewhere. Letting go in order to achieve something might seem strange. Yoga uses effort—doing—to aid surrender—undoing. With yoga you can often do more by undoing. As you release the air from your lungs, release the tension in the body. Don't force it. To extend farther, yield with each exhalation. Use rhythm to help you relax into the poses. If you have difficulty getting a sensation of release in a pose, use external movement. Move in and out of the pose with a rhythmic flow several times before holding the pose steady.

Finding the Edge

Learning to extend yourself to the limit requires experimentation to find just where the frontier lies. It changes daily, so you have to rediscover the edge in each pose of every practice. Metaphysically, reaching your edge and nudging your boundaries challenges your perception of where you are at. Yoga asanas are a controlled means of exposing yourself to a difficult situation. They are meant to try you. They offer practice at not being stressed in stressful conditions.

A single posture will have many edges. As you arrive at the first one, stay steady and breathe for a while. Have patience. Wait for the posture to let you in. When it does, enter respectfully. Again hold and breathe at this new edge, waiting for the invitation from your body to enter.

As you approach your "edge," distinguish between discomfort and pain. On the road to strength, flexibility, and focus, mental and physical unease inevitably arises. Discomfort is just resistance of the body or mind. Don't fight physical unease, but soften into it. For mental unease, become absorbed by the breath to return to the present.

Pain is more acute than discomfort. Pain in a pose means you have approached your edge too fast and gone too far or that you are improperly aligned. Pain in the muscles or joints should not be ignored because it can lead to injury. Come out of the pose and examine your alignment. Consult a teacher if necessary. In time you will become more body aware and better able to listen to feedback from your body.

Yoga is practicing being in the "now." Focus on your breathing to bring your attention to the present.

grounding

If you want one part of your body to rise up, you must anchor another part down. Each pose has an anchor point. Working from this base teaches you how to extend yourself, while not losing yourself. When no attention is given to grounding, yoga poses risk turning into a series of mere stretches.

Often less flexible people practice better yoga than very flexible ones, because stiffer-bodied people have more intuitive experience about anchoring and working from their bases. Very "stretchy" people sometimes find it hard to learn to anchor themselves. A certain amount of stability is always needed, both in life and in the poses. The earth supports, shelters, and feeds us, yet sometimes we lose our sense of connection with it. Re-center, find your balance, and extend yourself to your limit without losing awareness of what is always there to support you.

Resting

Nobody would expect an automobile driven continuously, at high speed, not to deteriorate. Yet many of us expect it from our bodies. Relaxation during asana practice allows the body space to give the mind feedback. Awareness and intuition will develop. Until the art of relaxation *within* the postures is developed, rest when necessary between postures. See Yoga Relaxation (pages 14–23) for resting poses.

There is a special quiet and receptive quality to the rest time between yoga postures.

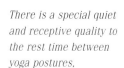

history and philosophy

Many scholars date Hatha yoga back to between the ninth and tenth centuries. However, the ideas and practices were passed down orally before being written down, so it is possible they are much older than this.

Yoga consists of eight limbs (see chart opposite), as codified in the *Yoga-Sutras*. Written in Sanskrit and attributed to Patanjali, the *Yoga-Sutras* is an early yoga text. Patanjali lists the eight limbs in a certain order, starting with moral behavior and ending with the self-realized state of samadhi.

They are not steps to be worked on one by one, but branches to be explored several at a time—otherwise we would forever remain at the very first precept of the first limb. Our whole lives would have to be lived without causing injury and we'd never move on to practicing a single asana.

From a relatively simple beginning using asanas, yoga sometimes takes you by the hand and leads you on to the higher concepts. You have the support of a force greater than yourself, so it feels like a natural progression to explore some of the other limbs.

The first five limbs are known as the outer limbs. Limbs three, four, and five involve the interpenetration of the mind, body, and spirit. The last three limbs, the inner limbs, are called the "wealth of yoga" by Patanjali. It's debatable whether you can "practice" them or not because they are states of the mind. However, you can make yourself as receptive as possible to them.

the eight limbs of yoga

1 *yama* Moral restraints. Five are listed in the Yoga-sutras: noninjury, truthfulness, nonstealing, chastity, and noncovetousness.

2 *niyama* Discipline in actions and conduct. Patanjali lists five disciplines: cleanliness, contentment, austerity, continuous learning, and surrender to the Divine.

3 *asana* The physical postures of Hatha yoga.

4 *pranayama* Breath control to cultivate the vital force within. For more information, see pages 28–30 and 104–116.

5 *pratyahara* Withdrawal of the senses. An example of pratyahara might be when you are so engrossed in watching a movie that you don't hear a fire truck siren outside. Often, instead of us controlling them, the senses become masters over us as we strive to satisfy our cravings. On the spiritual path, the mind gradually loses interest in what the senses have to say and pratyahara becomes more natural.

6 *dharana* Mental concentration. This can be practiced during asana and pranayama practice. Dharana helps pave the way to the seventh and eighth limbs. It is the third step in the practice in the section on Meditation.

7 *dhyana* As meditation, dhyana is a one-pointed mental focus (see pages 117–119).

8 *samadhi* Consciousness is altered in this illuminated state of absorption with the absolute.

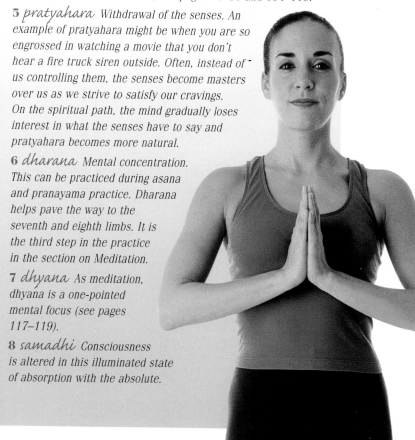

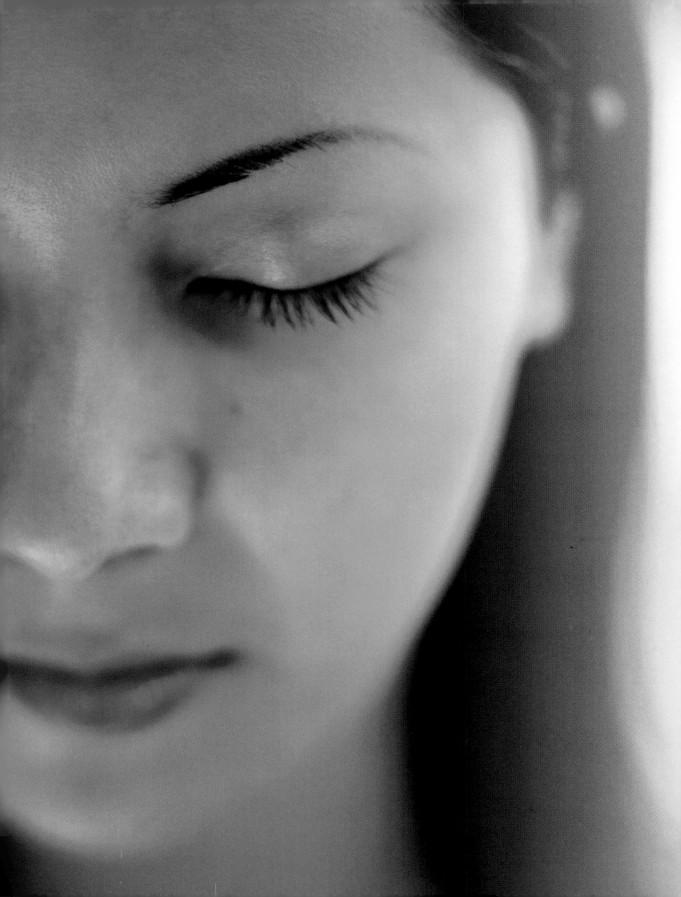

2 Yoga Relaxation

The role of deep relaxation in self-healing should never be underestimated. It is a generous act, not a selfish one, to give yourself restorative time. Relaxing fully lets you emerge refreshed and vibrant to participate in a wonderful, positive life. You will be better able to give more, live more, laugh more, and love more.

Deep relaxation teaches us how to let go. So often we cling on to objects, people, or ways of thinking. Relaxation is a time to withdraw from these attachments. Observe your thoughts, should they wander, then guide them gently back to the sensations of the body and let go of stored tension. In some ways deep relaxation is the most important part of the practice, so it should never be skipped.

center *yourself*

A short relaxation before starting and at the end of your asana practice will help you to center yourself. The final relaxation allows your body to integrate and consolidate the effects of the pose or poses you have been doing.

Imagine driving your automobile along the highway at 80 miles per hour, for weeks on end. What would happen if you stopped only briefly to check the oil and water and refill the fuel? How long would your automobile last if subjected to days, weeks, and years of this? Now consider how you are driving your body. Like your automobile, your body will run better if given high-quality fuel and regular tune-ups. It will perform better for you when allowed to cool down with regular rest breaks.

Yoga asanas stir up the subtle energies (prana) of the body and the relaxation is the time that allows the prana to be directed to healing and re-energizing the system. You might feel like nothing is happening and be tempted to skip this stage, but the final relaxation is hugely important and one risks losing valuable prana by missing it. Yoga relaxation allows you to emerge refreshed and brings your body, mind, and spirit back into balance. It is great after a long day or while recovering from illness. Taking a few minutes of conscious rest is enormously effective whenever you feel tired but need to keep working.

Many students gleefully exclaim "sleep" when relaxation time, *yoga nidra*, rolls around. Indeed, yoga nidra can be translated as "yogic sleep," but remember that it is a conscious rest, requiring discipline. You

practice being awake yet free of body tension. After a strong session where you have really explored your boundaries, this active undoing comes easier. As you take a break from external movement, cease fidgeting and lie perfectly still, the mind becomes acutely sensitive. While you progressively let go of tension in the muscles, bones, organs, even the brain, you remain aware of the internal sensations. Whenever your thoughts stray, bring them back to your body. As the senses quieten and attention is turned inward, there is a heightened awareness. Quietening the body and

Complete relaxation will come— it just takes practice.

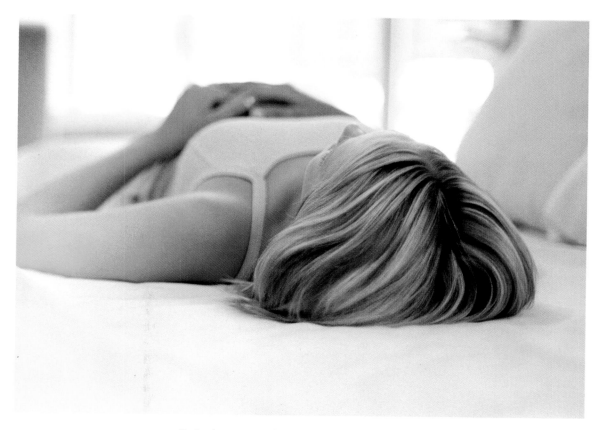

Notice how, as your body settles into yoga relaxation,
a feeling of expansion pervades.

mind, drawing the senses inward, and accessing your inner peace are steps along the path to meditation.

Lying still with your eyes closed looks easy. But if you tend to move through life at a frenetic pace, never ceasing to stop and take stock, falling into quietness can seem difficult. Conscious relaxation is an exercise in yielding. So many of us cling tenaciously to objects, people, habits, or attitudes. The principle of detachment is fundamental to Eastern philosophies. While you remain strongly attached to things, their loss will inevitably cause suffering. If you observe yourself holding onto things and accumulating material possessions, use yoga relaxation consciously to practice letting go. Physically and mentally permit yourself to release that grip and be just you, nothing else, lying on the floor. As you actively undo, you let your defenses down and accept the sense of vulnerability inherent in allowing surrender.

Try making a fist with one hand and keeping it clenched for ten seconds. Now relax the fist and compare the feelings in the two hands. Most likely you'll feel more sensations in the hand that was clenched. As you seek to find the edge in each posture, you will be fully occupying both muscles and mind. Once the tension is released, a lingering awareness remains. The same principle applies in yoga relaxation. When you have extended your body to its limit, you'll notice how your awareness of internal sensations deepens because your mind has been completely engrossed in your practice. It will very easily let go into deep relaxation.

One necessary word of warning: if you suffer from depression or phobias, don't practice Savasana without expert guidance and supervision.

getting comfortable for *relaxation*

Help yourself let go by becoming perfectly physically comfortable. Any of these modifications to the basic supine position may be helpful. See page 22 for how to make a breathing bed. Child Pose (see page 19) is useful whenever you need to relax during your practice or at any point during the day.

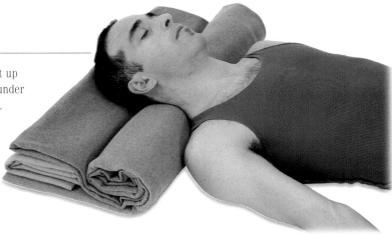

Making a Neck Pillow

Fold a blanket three times and roll it up about halfway. Wedge this securely under your neck, right up to shoulder level. Experiment with the amount of roll. Your neck should feel very snug with the roll supporting its natural curve. Usually the chin juts out a little. If this is so, fold the remaining flap down to cushion and lift the back of the head.

Your chin and forehead should ideally be at equal height from the floor.

Using a Pillow

Find the best position for your head by having a friend observe you as you lie on your back. Ideally, your chin and forehead will be at equal heights from the floor. If your chin is higher than your forehead the back of the neck will tend to shorten. Many people don't need more than a thinly folded blanket to soften the floor for the head. However, if you find your chin juts up higher than your forehead when you are lying, make a pillow.

If the forehead is too high, the throat will feel constricted. Use a folded blanket to bring your chin and forehead level.

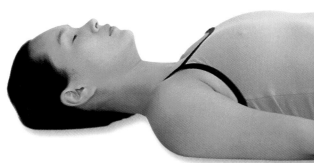

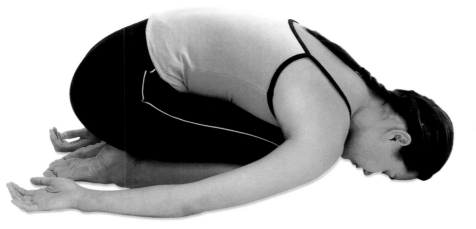

Use Child Pose whenever you need to relax. This simple posture can help you connect to feelings of safety and trust.

Supporting the Lower Back

This support lets the lower back soften down closer to the floor, and those with lower back problems find it useful. Place large rolled cushions or a bolster under your knees, and do a small pelvic tilt to flatten the lower back toward the floor. Your lower back will still curve up away from the floor, but as you then lie and let go, you will feel it ease out and release a little. If you don't have any props, then bend your knees up, place your feet just wider than body width, and lean the knees in together.

Child Pose—Balasana

Sit on your heels with your knees together. Fold forward over your thighs. Rest your forehead on the floor and drape your arms around you. Close your eyes and let go of any tension. Enjoy the reassuring massage of the belly pressing down into the thighs with each inhalation. For high blood pressure, or if your buttocks stay high in the air and you feel like you are nosediving, rest the forehead on a pad of folded blankets. Alternatively, stack your fists and rest your forehead on them.

Try experimenting with different levels of padding under the knees.

cover up

When you relax deeply, your body temperature drops dramatically. It is impossible to completely let go when you are cold. Unless it is the height of summer, cover your whole body with a shawl or blanket when practicing relaxing.

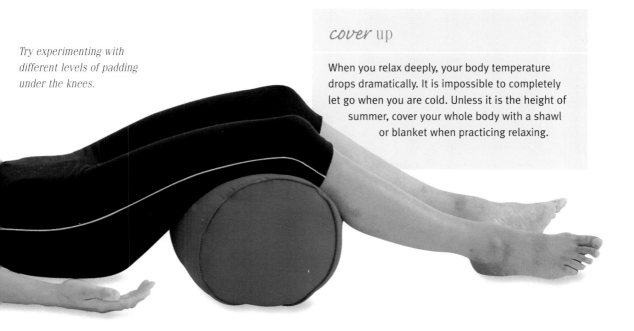

guided relaxation in
savasana corpse pose

While this pose looks like the easiest of all the yoga asanas, it is actually one of the hardest to master. While the body lets go, the mind must stay alert, observing the relaxation process, before finally surrendering into rest. The final relaxation allows your body to settle and the effects of your Hatha yoga practice to consolidate. Spend five or ten minutes working through the body to exaggerate the tension in your muscles, section by section. This raises the level of awareness so you can better surrender into complete relaxation. A nice way to practice Savasana is to make a tape of these instructions, with plenty of pauses, or have a friend read them aloud.

1 Lie on your back in Savasana. Your legs are apart with feet rolling out to the sides. Your arms are just out from your sides. Have the backs of your hands on the floor so your fingers curl softly up. Close your eyes so attention is drawn inward and you become sensitized to your inner environment.

2 Scrunch your toes and flex your feet. Next, spread out your toes and point the feet strongly. Then relax your feet.

3 Lift your right leg 2 in (5 cm) in the air. Briefly tense all the muscles in that leg, then release them, letting the leg fall to the floor. Do the same with the left leg.

4 Clench your buttocks for a few seconds so your hips rise up slightly. Release. Feel the heaviness of your lower body.

5 Tighten the muscles along the length of the spine and press the tips of your shoulders into the floor. Puff your chest up and tighten your abdominal muscles. Then exhale and relax the muscles, let the chest release down, and allow the tension to flow out of the body.

6 Lift one arm 2 in (5 cm) off the ground. Tighten all its muscles, make a fist with your hand, then stretch the fingers out. Exhale and let all the tension go so the arm drops back down on the floor. Repeat on the other side.

7 Lift the shoulders to the ears in a shrug and then release them back down and toward the hips.

8 Tighten all the facial muscles. Lose your inhibitions—no one is watching you! Clench your jaw muscles, squeeze the eyes tightly shut, and frown. Then widen everything out and apart. Open your eyes and roll the eyeballs back, open your mouth and stick the tongue as far out toward the chin as you can. Finally, exhale with a sigh and relax the face. Feel all the skin on the face soften and any wrinkles smooth out.

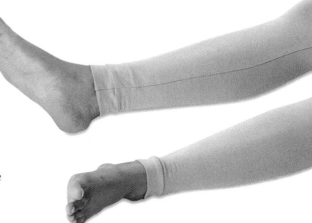

9 This time without tensing, gently drop your right ear to the floor. Take a few long breaths and become aware of the stretch on the left side of the neck. Inhale, the head to the center, and drop the left ear to the floor for a few breaths before bringing the head to center again.

10 Press the chin to the throat so you feel the back of the neck lengthening, then release it by softening all the neck muscles. So that you can commit to lying perfectly still for the next 10 minutes, mentally check your position and adjust anything you need to. Just as during meditation, any outer movement will distract you from your inner world.

11 Become aware of the whole body being heavy and relaxed. Your body wants to be comfortable. It is its natural state. The bones feel heavy. All the muscles are relaxed. The internal organs are free of tension. Even the tongue is relaxed. As the body releases and feels heavier, the breath lightens and feels more delicate. The brain surrenders any worries and is content, enjoying this peaceful and tranquil moment. Give permission for your emotional body to let go too. While the body relaxes, the mind stays present, observing. Finally, completely stop trying to "do." Let go of any psychological effort at all. Now rest.

12 You will intuitively know when it's time to come out of the relaxation. Begin to move the fingers and toes as you focus back on the body. Take your arms overhead along the floor and stretch up through the body, enlivening everything from fingertips to toes. When you are ready, roll over onto your side and allow the eyes to open in their own time.

explore *yoga*

You don't need to practice any asanas to reward yourself with Savasana. Practice relaxation whenever you feel tired. Instead of taking a daytime nap, refresh with 10 minutes of Savasana.

However, if you occasionally have time to combine your asana exercises into a longer session, practice at least 5 minutes of Savasana for every 30 minutes of asana practice. For a 90-minute practice, allow 15 minutes of relaxation at the end.

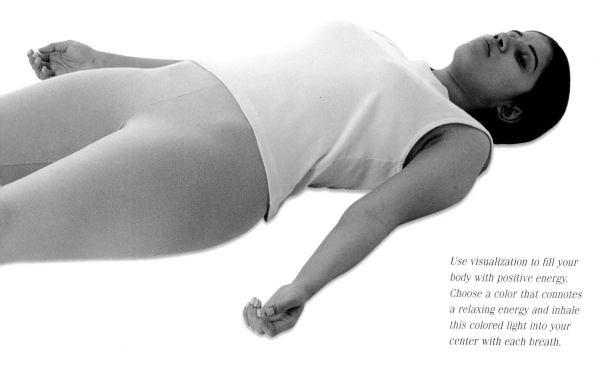

Use visualization to fill your body with positive energy. Choose a color that connotes a relaxing energy and inhale this colored light into your center with each breath.

revitalizing *relaxation*

To make a breathing bed, fold one to three blankets so they are 8 in (20 cm) wide and longer than your torso. Lie over them with your buttocks on the floor and legs a little apart. The more blankets you use, the more the chest will feel it is opening, so experiment with what feels best for you. Use another blanket as a pillow so that the head is higher than the chest. Take your legs apart and let your arms rest out to the sides.

Lie on your back and lift your head for a moment to look down your body to make sure that you are perfectly symmetrical. After checking that you feel completely comfortable, begin to breathe deeply and rhythmically. As you inhale, visualize prana being drawn in through the nostrils down to your solar plexus. As you exhale it swirls around your center. With each inhalation, draw this pranic energy down to the solar plexus so that it spirals around filling up the whole torso. Each long, deep inhalation draws in more prana. While you are giving yourself the gift of vibrant energy, remember to keep the exhalations slow and steady. The full exhalation empties the lungs, allowing you to inhale this revitalizing force deeply and consciously.

From the center of the torso the spiral enlarges to cover the whole body. The outer part of the spiral reaches to circle over the head, fingertips, and toes. Let yourself become the breath. With this positive energy you become enthusiastic about life and your tasks. You gain the energy to fulfil them. Stay here as long as you feel you need to.

When it is time to awaken, start moving your body gently and begin to stretch a little. Feel so revitalized that the eyes blink open by themselves, as if powered by the new energy within.

When it is time to come back, rouse yourself from sitting and take the journey back until you see yourself lying on the floor again. Tune in to your surroundings, then roll over and sit up slowly.

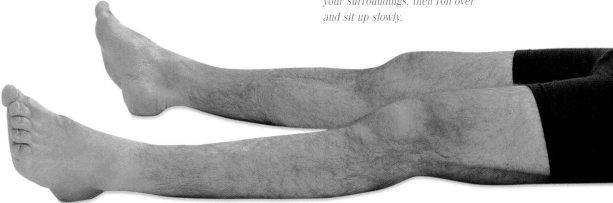

relaxation *visualization*

Creating a Sanctuary

Think of a place where you know you can feel completely at ease. It could be a real place you have visited or seen or else an imaginary paradise—a special sanctuary where you feel completely safe, protected and nurtured. It might be next to a still, deep pond, near the ocean, in a lush green forest, or by a flickering fireplace in a wonderful home. Now, as you lie in Savasana, visualize yourself from above. From lying on the floor, visualize your body coming up to standing, and start on a pleasant trip toward your special place. Feel the sun on your skin and the breeze in your hair. Listen to the call of the birds and the other sounds around like leaves in the gentle wind or a babbling brook. In time, you arrive at your special place and settle yourself down to sit in a meditative position. Visualize yourself sitting with eyes closed and peaceful mind. Your sanctuary gives you nourishment, and you are safe there to relax completely. Continue to see yourself sitting quietly. Know that your sanctuary is always there whenever you need it. You just need to take the time to access it.

When it is time to come back, rouse yourself from sitting and take the journey back to where you are lying, until you can see yourself on the floor again. Begin to tune in to the sounds around you once again. Feel the touch of the clothes on your skin, then roll over and sit up slowly.

explore *yoga*

To stay true to your inner self and to protect yourself from being harmed or feeling drained by other people, visualize yourself surrounded with glowing white light.

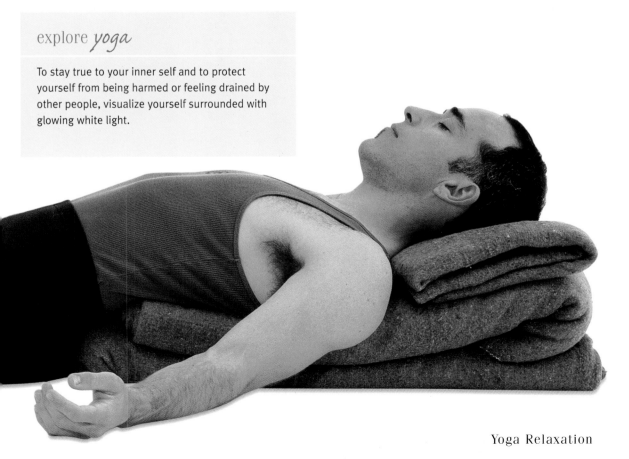

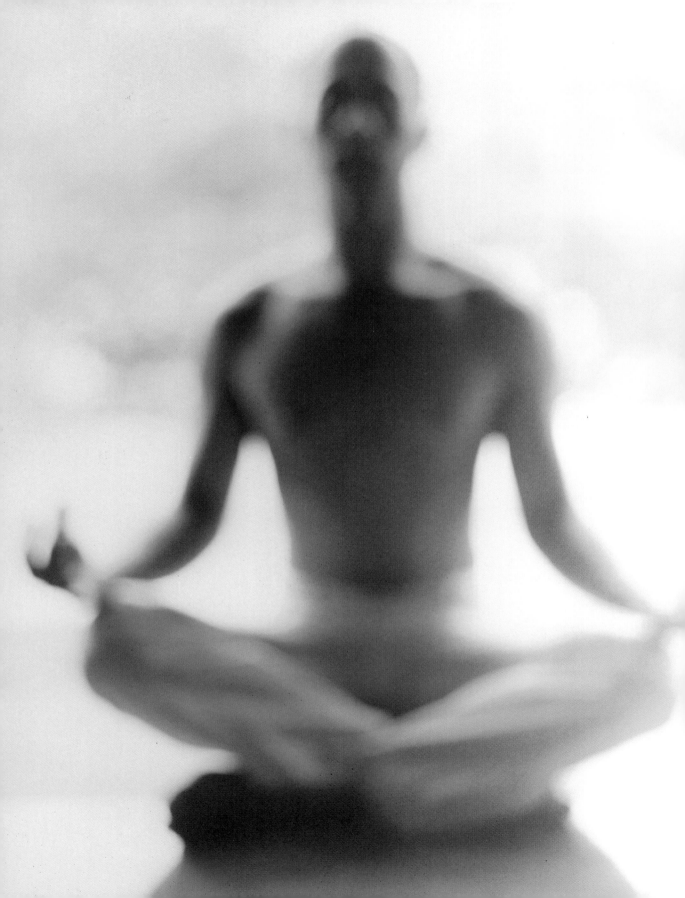

3 ThePractice

Creating a special yoga practice area will reaffirm your commitment. You don't need much space, but make sure the area is warm, clean, and uncluttered. Choose non-restrictive clothes that you feel good in. Dress in layers to remain comfortable throughout your practice. Bare feet are best—wear socks only when your feet are cold. Intense practice in direct sunlight tends to be fatiguing, but relaxing in its warmth at the end is lovely. Practicing outside lets you commune with nature, but it can be more distracting than staying inside. It's a great idea to invest in a yoga mat. Apart from providing cushioning and a non-slip surface, it will make your mental commitment to your practice stronger. You will feel you can create a yoga space anywhere, simply by rolling out your mat.

starting the *journey*

The following guidelines will help you get more out of your practice. Remember, never rush your yoga practice. More benefit is derived from spending 10 minutes on just a few postures than skipping through an entire routine quickly and with less awareness.

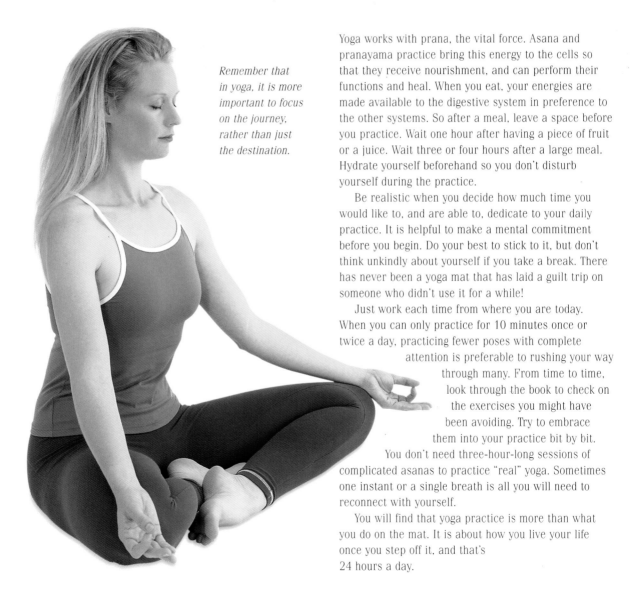

Remember that in yoga, it is more important to focus on the journey, rather than just the destination.

Yoga works with prana, the vital force. Asana and pranayama practice bring this energy to the cells so that they receive nourishment, and can perform their functions and heal. When you eat, your energies are made available to the digestive system in preference to the other systems. So after a meal, leave a space before you practice. Wait one hour after having a piece of fruit or a juice. Wait three or four hours after a large meal. Hydrate yourself beforehand so you don't disturb yourself during the practice.

Be realistic when you decide how much time you would like to, and are able to, dedicate to your daily practice. It is helpful to make a mental commitment before you begin. Do your best to stick to it, but don't think unkindly about yourself if you take a break. There has never been a yoga mat that has laid a guilt trip on someone who didn't use it for a while!

Just work each time from where you are today. When you can only practice for 10 minutes once or twice a day, practicing fewer poses with complete attention is preferable to rushing your way through many. From time to time, look through the book to check on the exercises you might have been avoiding. Try to embrace them into your practice bit by bit.

You don't need three-hour-long sessions of complicated asanas to practice "real" yoga. Sometimes one instant or a single breath is all you will need to reconnect with yourself.

You will find that yoga practice is more than what you do on the mat. It is about how you live your life once you step off it, and that's 24 hours a day.

There are thousands of variations on hundreds of yoga poses but don't let this intimidate you. Even if you feel like a human ironing board, you can benefit enormously from about 20 poses practiced regularly. It's like tending a garden. Left uncared for, the soil starts to dry up and the plants start to wither. Once the garden has gotten to a certain state, it's too late to rush in with the big hoses. Large amounts of water might be more than it can readily accept, and instead it needs the kindness of water given little and often. If you have neglected your internal garden for a while, you'll need to practice in small, regular doses for it to grow and begin to thrive.

Rather than focus on "perfecting" a posture as your measure of success in yoga, enjoy discovering your body and mind. Yoga is like life. It's a journey. You will find that every yoga practice you have will be different, as you respond to internal and external conditions. Your thoughts change in a fraction of a second. The breath alters from second to second. How far you can stretch or hold a pose changes from minute to minute.

Empty your mind so that you can fully absorb the lessons of your practice. You never can predict just what they will be. If you are more adept, don't assume because you have practiced a posture a hundred times that you know everything about it. Keep the mind receptive and open to learning. Don't be impatient in your practice. Practice peacefully. Keep your mind sensitive. Overstraining the body will lessen your mental sensitivity. Some days you just might not feel like getting on your mat or doing breath work. Instead, your yoga practice on these occasions might include reading something spiritually uplifting.

Take things easy during menstruation. It's a special time when it is nice to allow your energies to go inside. Avoid strong backbends and strong twists. Inverted postures make the flow have to work against gravity so avoid them. Women have a natural body clock that reminds them to practice slow, restful yoga regularly, but in my classes, men are allowed to "menstruate" too! See the therapeutic yoga section (pages 122–127) for more information.

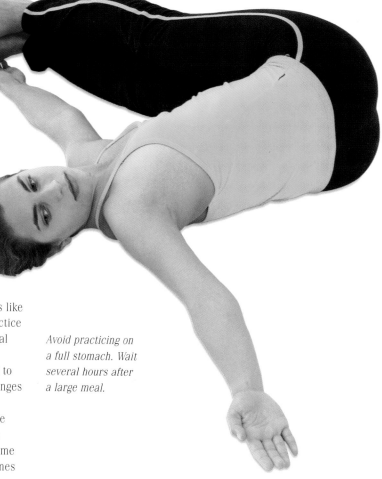

Avoid practicing on a full stomach. Wait several hours after a large meal.

While yoga has helped the pregnancies and labors of countless women, it is not safe to begin during the first three months of pregnancy. Many poses need to be modified so it's best to attend specialized classes during the second and third trimesters. See the section on therapeutic yoga for more information.

If you are suffering from any kind of health condition or have an injury, seek guidance from an experienced yoga teacher or yoga therapist. Don't practice asanas or pranayama if you have a fever.

If you have the time, attend some yoga classes. Yoga is so personal that each teacher will have something different to offer you. Teachers can give valuable feedback on your alignment and ideas for practice. Try teachers from several different traditions of yoga to find which kind suits you best.

awareness of the *breath*

Lie on your back with your knees bent and feet flat on the floor. Swivel your feet so your big toes are closer together than your inner heels, then lean your knees in together so that holding them in place is effortless. Have your arms out by your sides, palms facing down. Close your eyes. Give your full attention to your breathing.

Can you feel where the breath originates? Observe which part of your body moves first as you breathe in. What happens next? Observe the sequence of your body's movement when you inhale. Feel what happens to the lower and upper abdomen. How do the rib cage and chest work? Can you feel anything happening at the back? What happens to the shoulders, throat, face, and nostrils? Does anything change at the area of the pelvis?

Absorb yourself completely in your breath. You are your breath and your breath is you. It rises and falls with the rhythm of ocean waves. How do you accept your inhalation? How do you feel the expansion?

Now turn your attention to the out breath. From where do you exhale? Which part of the body begins the movement? Where does your exhalation end? Are the

movements in the torso as clearly demarcated as in your inhalation? Can you feel a consolidation of energy? Accept the support of the earth with each breath. Don't shrink, but let yourself sink.

Count the length of your in and out breaths. Which is longer? Does one come more easily to you? Become aware of the quality of your breath. Is it shallow or deep? How rhythmic does it feel? Does it feel smooth or coarse? Is it graceful and round, or are there some parts that feel jerky or jagged? Does it feel soothing?

Often we don't breathe out fully, but hurry on to the next inhalation. Take the time to follow the entire length of your exhalation. Stay with it. Patiently wait until it is finished before you take your next breath. It takes some time to release all the used air from the alveoli. There is no need to tighten any muscles to "squeeze" the last air out. Just be patient and let it keep on flowing. Whenever you feel you are trying too hard, release the effort.

Concentrating on your breathing leads to a new sense of awareness, and calms the mind.

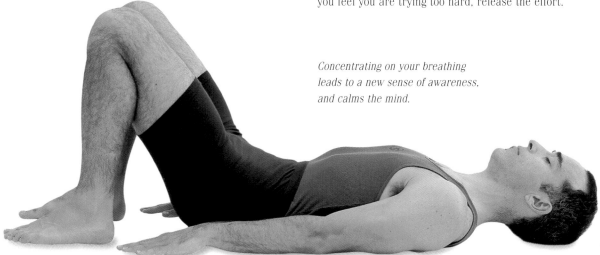

Now become aware of the time at the end of the exhalation before the next inhalation begins. There is a brief moment before your lungs call for air. Don't grab for the next breath. Sink into this natural pause and enjoy it. It is a moment of tranquility, as still as a deep, calm pond. The exhalation disappears into it, and then the stillness gives birth to the inhalation. As you observe this stillness, you may find the pause lengthening naturally.

Now attune yourself to what happens at the top of the inhalation, before you feel the need to exhale. There is another pause, another precious moment. It is a full silence that you can relax into. As you let yourself sink into this moment it will expand.

These pauses give rise to a breath in four parts: a releasing exhalation, a still pause, the gift of a new inhalation, and a pause. Become absorbed in a meditative way in each part of your breath. No two breaths are the same. Make friends with your breathing and get to know each part intimately.

Before you roll over to sit up, take some time to observe the effects this exercise has had on your mind. You have learned a new skill to quieten the mind. You will find you have developed your self-awareness, and practiced being absorbed in the present moment.

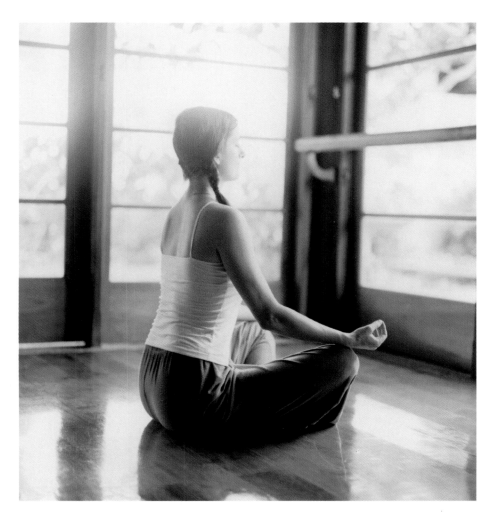

Learn to enjoy the stillness of the natural pause between an out breath and the next inhalation, and again before exhaling.

chest opening exercise

Channeling the breath into movement is centering and helps maintain a steady, rhythmic breath. Quieten the mind and observe the present moment by focusing on your breath.

1 Lie on your back with your knees bent up and your hands palms-down on the floor. To begin, exhale fully.

2 While you inhale, raise your arms up and overhead until the backs of your hands come to rest on or near the floor. Energize your arms so that they extend and lift out of your shoulders to flow through a large arc.

3 Exhale and raise your arms up to bring them back to the starting position. With eyes closed, continue moving between these two movements. Time the movement to follow your breath, not the other way around. Because you keep the flow of air in and out through the nostrils at a steady rate, your arm movements are also constant, rhythmic and graceful.

4 Now become aware of how your torso moves in relation to the arm movements. As you inhale and raise the arms up, feel the natural life of the upper back as it lifts away from the floor. Rest with your arms overhead for several breaths. The upper back will ground more into the floor and your chest will naturally open and promote a satisfyingly full inhalation. Each time you exhale and bring your arms down, tune into the softening down that happens in the torso as it releases into the earth. Moving slowly, with awareness, bring your attention to your pelvis. Can you feel the gentle tilting back and forward with each part of the breath?

Take some more time, unhurriedly observing the movements of the body in response to the breath.

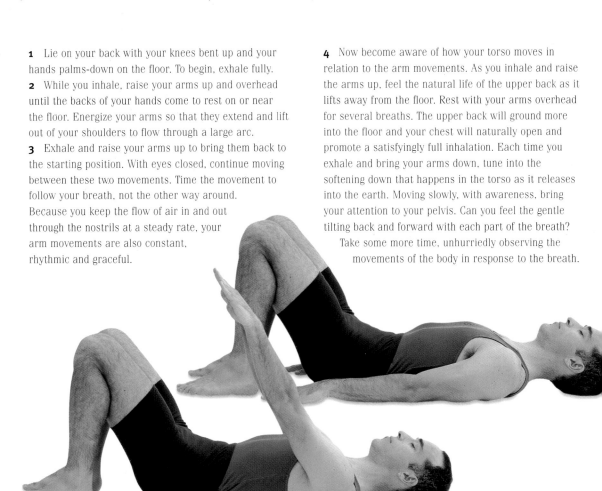

cat pose
biralasana

This exercise brings awareness and flexibility to the entire length of the spine. The key to awareness is to move slowly. Practice patience and keep an inquiring mind.

1 Begin on all fours with your knees under your hips and your hands just forward of your shoulders.

2 Inhale and concave your back. Move your breastbone forward and up and raise your tailbone. Keep the back of your neck long as you gaze upward. Pressurize the palms evenly against the floor. Avoid slumping into the shoulders.

3 As you exhale, round your back. Your upper back arches naturally in this way, so place particular awareness on the movement of the lower back as it follows this new curve upward as you tuck your pelvis under. Observe how your shoulder blades spread apart and the skin between them stretches. As you finish your exhalation, move your chin toward your breastbone.

4 Repeat ten more rounds, arching and rounding in time to your breath. Accentuate the curve in the repeats so that it is deeper each time.

explore*yoga*

The vertebral column is made up of 33 vertebrae. The bottom nine are fused, but the remaining 24 are not. Try to narrow your focus to a single vertebra at a time. Mentally go inside to observe its range of movement. Alternatively, begin the movement at the tailbone and concave your back, moving vertebra by vertebra, up the spine, taking as many breaths as you need to complete the movement.

roll downs

Working through this sequence will allow you to learn about how undoing, rather than active doing, can deepen a pose.

1 Stand in Tadasana (see page 40) with your feet hip-width apart. You are going to take several breaths to fold forward by rolling down the spine.

2 As you exhale, drop your head forward. Feel how the shoulders want to follow. Release your knees so that they bend slightly. On your next exhalation let the shoulders go and the upper back round more. Your arms hang down vertically, dangling passively out of their sockets. Continue exhaling and rolling down the back in stages, leading with the head. Your knees will bend more the further you roll down. Take as many breaths as you need to release all the way down.

3 Even though your legs are working, your upper body is dangling, hanging out of the hips. Bring a rag-doll quality to the upper body. Move your awareness to the shoulders and relax them fully so that the arms hang loose. Relax the back of the neck so that the crown of the head is the closest part of the head to the floor.

4 Take several rounds of breathing, observing the movements intrinsically related to the breath. As you inhale there is a lifting energy in the core of the body. If your knees are bent enough, a small lengthening occurs from pubic bone to throat. As you exhale your ribs will fall closer to your thighs.

5 When it's time to come up, keep the knees bent and, over several breaths, roll up slowly through the spine, as if you are stacking each vertebra on top of the last. Exhale; release the arms down to the sides.

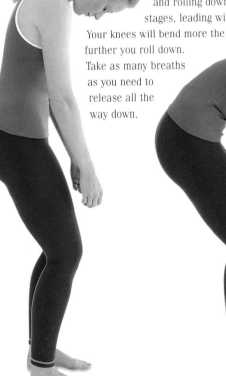
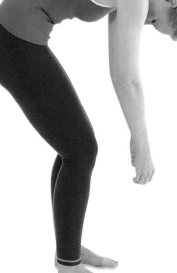
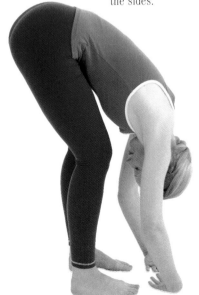

cross-legged forward fold
sukhasana forward fold

Sukha means content or happy. Spend a few minutes letting yourself soften into this pose as a centering way to start your practice.

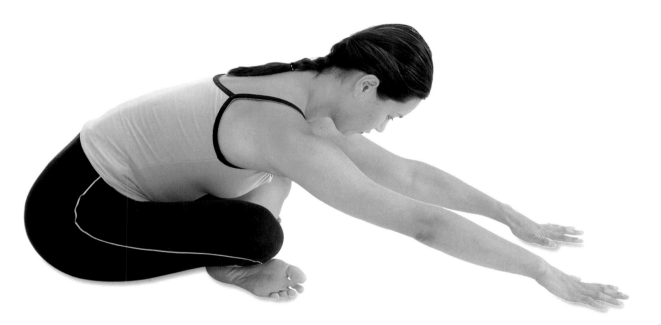

1 Begin by sitting in a simple cross-legged position. To work deeper into the hips, slide your heels away from each other so that they are resting under the opposite knees. Then take the feet forward so that the shins are in a horizontal line.

2 Become aware of the sitting bones in contact with the floor. This base will act as your anchor as you stretch forward. Place your fingertips on the floor just in front of your legs. Now lengthen the sides of the torso from hips to armpits. Use several breaths to let this releasing take place. When you feel ready, creep the hands away. Work with your breath as you take one or two minutes to slide the hands forward in stages. Only drop your forehead down to the floor if your front ribs come to lie on your legs. Then repeat with the legs crossed the other way.

explore *yoga*

Don't become mentally lazy. Stay aware. If you are simply performing the pose automatically, you may well just stay at the point you initially reached. When you use longer holds in a pose, often you will find you can go much deeper and gradually extend yourself to your new edge.

sun salutation

surya namaskar

The Sun Salutation is a group of postures that flow together to warm the body and work the heart. While you link movement and breath, you stretch and strengthen the muscles, developing stamina, coordination, and confidence. There are many possible variations of Surya Namaskar to suit all ages and abilities, so ask a yoga teacher for help if necessary.

1 Mountain Pose With palms together, ground through the feet and feel the connection with the earth through the soles of the feet.

11 Switch on your thigh muscles and those of the lower abdomen as you inhale skyward. Lift everything from the hips up, except the shoulders.

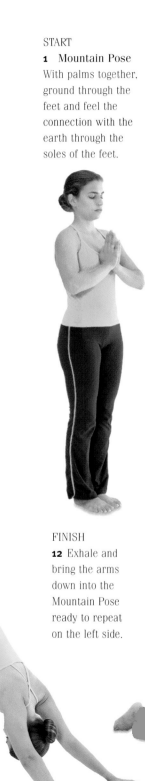

10 Intense Forward Stretch Exhale as you step your left leg forward to fold the body down over your legs. If your legs are straight, press your hands more to the floor.

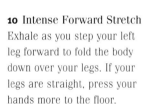

FINISH **12** Exhale and bring the arms down into the Mountain Pose ready to repeat on the left side.

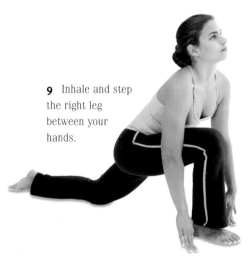

9 Inhale and step the right leg between your hands.

8 Downward-Facing Dog Exhale while you tuck your toes under and lift the hips high. Hold for three breaths.

2 Inhale and take your arms skyward. As the front of your torso lengthens, keep the back side of the torso long as well.

3 Intense Forward Stretch Exhale and fold forward to touch the earth.

The sun is a symbol of the inner light that is in all of us. The bowing is an exercise of deep respect for this shining light; the folding and unfolding movements a tribute to creation. As you develop a graceful flow of one movement per breath, it becomes a moving meditation. Start your practice with three rounds and build to six, offering each one up like a prayer. Then sit quietly and listen as your body tells you what it would like to practice next.

explore*yoga*

Give yourself time to feel your way into the poses by holding each one for several slow breaths. Practice Ujjayi breathing (see page 113) during the Sun Salutation.

4 With fingertips touching the floor (bend your knees if necessary), lunge. Inhale and step your right leg back. Lift your chest away from your thighs.

7 Cobra Lower your body to the floor, then inhale as you press your hands to the floor to curve the chest up in Cobra Pose.

6 Still exhaling, bring your shoulders forward of your wrists, so your elbows form a right angle as you lower your body to 2 in (5 cm) off the floor.

5 Exhale and step your feet back to plank pose, forming a straight line from heels to shoulders.

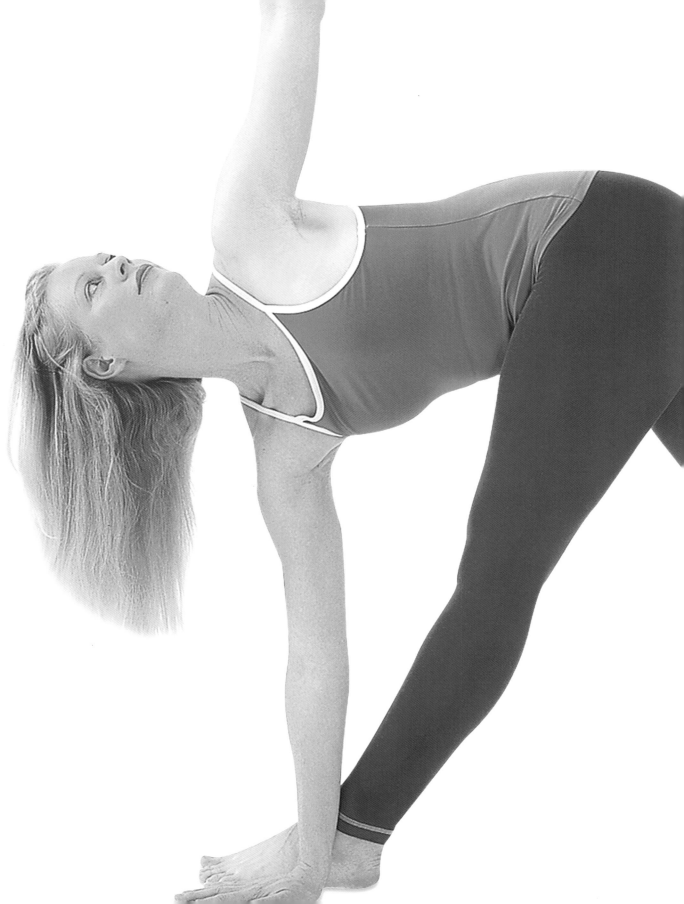

4 Standing Postures

Regular practice of the standing poses is a great start for all yogis as they increase strength and flexibility in equal parts. Since they extend and integrate the whole body, they help correct imbalances of the vertebral column. They develop grace, endurance, perseverance, and concentration. They also help you to feel more energetic and enthusiastic.

Since they involve the whole body, standing poses warm you in preparation for the other poses, making a good start to any yoga practice.

In order to achieve anything in life, we need somewhere to extend from. Standing postures let us develop roots. They allow us to examine how we "stand on our own two feet" and how to "stand our ground." In learning to "stand tall" we are able to achieve our full height. They help us establish a firm base to ensure that the upper body is well supported. In standing poses we play off stability with extension as we practice radiating outward from this steady base.

about *alignment*

Your feet need to be well aligned in order to bring good posture to the rest of the body. Stand with your feet a little less than hip-width apart. Feel free to experiment to find the width that gives you the most centered feeling.

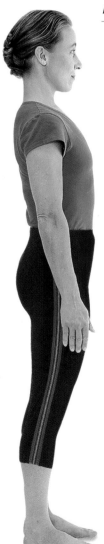

From the Ground Up

1 Have a good look at your feet. How are the arches? Do they lift up like little rainbows, or do they collapse downward to produce flat feet or knock-knees? How are your toes? Are they squashed together from years of wearing tight shoes? Are they white with tension as they cling to the ground? Ungrip the toes by lifting them up and spreading them apart. Keeping them stretched away, place them down on the floor.

2 Stand erect once more and feel where the heaviness comes into the feet. Where is the weight centered? Is there more weight placed on the ball of the feet, or the heels? Is one foot taking more weight than another? Rock back and forth to find your center. Keeping the feet on the floor, transfer the weight from left to right several times to home in on the center of grounding. Lean in all directions in a large circle. Then slowly reduce the size of the circle until you come to find your centered point.

3 Mentally soften the soles of your feet. Spread the skin. Let your breath come into the feet. They widen and soften with each exhalation. Visualize roots growing downward. By earthing the feet, the rest of the body is free to expand and lengthen.

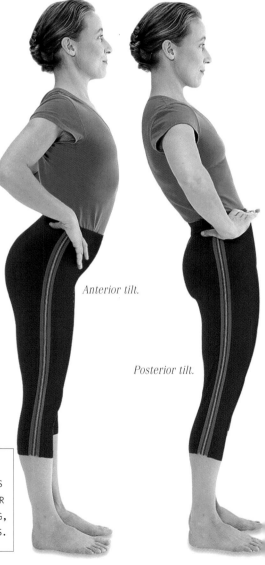

Anterior tilt.

Posterior tilt.

> AVOID STANDING POSES IN ACUTE CASES OF ASTHMA, COLITIS, NERVOUS DISORDERS OR CARDIAC PROBLEMS. DON'T JUMP IN OR OUT OF THE POSES IF YOU ARE MENSTRUATING, PREGNANT, OR HAVE BACK OR KNEE INJURIES.

From the Pelvis Up

1 Anterior tilt. Stand with your hands on your hips, fingers pointing forward, so that your index fingers rest on top of the hipbones and press into the waist. Pelvis means "basin" in Latin. Tilt your pelvis forward, just as if it were a basin and you were tipping water out of the front of it. Your fingers will point down and your thumbs will lift up. Feel how the curve in your lower back accentuates and your chest lifts a bit. This action makes the knees push back too.

2 Posterior tilt. Now tilt the pelvis the other way, as if you were pouring out water from the back. Your fingers will rise up and your thumbs move down. Observe how this changes your posture. Your lower back curve will flatten and the fronts of your knees will move forward. The chest tends to slump, abdominal length shortens, and shoulders roll forward. Feel how this affects your neck too. If you are not sure, exaggerating the movements might help make the dynamic clearer.

3 Come back to the center, so your pelvis is not tipped forward or back, but centered. Take time to feel how it is, mentally comparing it to your normal way of standing. By taking time to move in between the anterior and posterior pelvic tilt positions, you will become familiar with the trickle-on effects of them both on the rest of your body. A truly centered pelvis would actually be too unstable to carry us well, so people tend to have a pelvis tilted either one way or the other. Ideally this position would be just off center, rather than strongly so.

Still standing, find a more centered position for your pelvis. Take time to scan through your body, observing how it feels when comparing it to your normal way of carrying yourself. Slowly move around the room like this, exploring some new possibilities for your carriage and movement.

explore*yoga*

Stay in your habitual standing position without moving for long enough for the sensations to intensify. Then take this feedback and see what you need to do to realign and prevent the discomfort coming to those points.

Elongating the Curves of the Spine

1 Stand with your back to the corner of a wall or the edge of a doorframe. Take your feet about 1 ft (30 cm) away from the wall, and a little bit apart, with the outside edges of the feet parallel. Lean against the wall so that your body contacts the wall at the sacrum and the thoracic curve. The small of the back (lumbar region) will arch away from the wall. How easily the back of your head comes to the wall depends on the curves of your spine. If your upper back is very flat, your throat will feel constricted. If your upper back is very rounded, it will be more difficult to bring your head comfortably to the wall. If your chin juts out and the back of the neck shortens, find a midway position for the head. Gently bring your floating ribs down, so that they don't jut out. Don't bend your knees. Now bring the tops of the thighs back slightly so that the front of the groin opens.

2 The spine is most effectively lengthened by undoing, rather than doing. Take plenty of time to release so that the spine can elongate upward. If you actively work the muscles that run along the spine then they will contract and actually shorten the vertebral column. Likewise, there is no need to raise the shoulders up to grow taller. Instead, let go with each exhalation. Let your tailbone be heavy so it eases down toward the floor. Keep your weight well grounded through your feet. As you continue to lengthen, feel the very small movements that ripple along the spine in connection with the breath. Are there any areas of your spine that feel blocked? Concentrate on softening the tight spots. When you move away from the wall, walk softly around the room feeling the effects of this exercise.

mountain pose
tadasana

This pose connects you to both earth and sky. It is a wonderful exercise in centering and being able to respond to situations from a solid base. Begin and end each of the standing poses with this centered position. Use it as a chance to hear your body's feedback to what happened in the last pose. Although you appear steady as a mountain, you are not as hard as a rock in this pose. Externally your mountain is still, but bring it alive from the inside, where it feels dynamic and alive, responding to every breath. Practice Tadasana whenever you have a free moment during the day.

1 Stand with your feet a little less than hip-width apart, with the insides of your feet parallel. Follow the instructions for softening the feet on page 38. While your feet ground downward, move your awareness to your legs and get a sense of extending up toward the sky, starting at the ankle joints. Let your pelvis be in a neutral position (see previous page). The spine, supported by the pelvis, is freed to lengthen upward. It is perfectly possible to stand erect and be relaxed at the same time. Exhale tension out of the spine so it is released to grow taller. Get a sense of your arms dangling from the shoulder sockets. Let them just hang, and completely let go. As your shoulders soften down, the neck and head float and rise up out of them. Release the mouth, tongue, and jaw. Observe whether this allows other more distant parts of the body to release too. Bring a sense of weightlessness to the head by visualizing it as a helium-filled balloon attached to the end of a stick, your spine. Mentally sweep over your body to see where the heaviness is.

2 Check in with your breathing. Release the diaphragm muscle. Take slow, deep, steady breaths. Feel the ripple-like effect of each breath on the spine. Quite different from an upward movement induced by muscle tension, feel the lifting energy with each inhalation. Your body has its own innate intelligence. Be curious! Follow your breath to feel where it lets your body open and expand. Explore any subtle effects that your exhalation has on it.

warrior I
virabhadrasana I

This all-involving pose works the arms and legs, strengthens the back, and opens the chest.

1   Stand with your legs about 4 ft (1.2 m) apart. Turn your whole right leg and foot deeply inward 60 degrees. Turn your left leg and foot out 90 degrees and swivel your whole upper body so it faces over your left leg. Open the groin by letting your left hip move forward to align with the right. If this is difficult, turn the back leg and foot in deeper. An easier alternative is to have the feet parallel and lift the back heel up a little off the floor (see right).

2   Bend your left knee to a 90-degree angle. Keep your back leg straight by pressing the back heel away to open the back of the knee.

3   Take your arms out to the sides, turn the palms up, and raise the arms overhead to join the palms. Gaze at your thumbs. Stretch up from the hips to the fingertips. As you breathe deeply, feel the stretch of skin on the chest and abdomen. Stay for ten breaths, and maintain perfect awareness as you come out of the pose and move to the right side.

Alternative

An easier alternative for beginners is to have the feet parallel and lift the back heel off the floor. If you have trouble balancing, step the front foot a little to the side. Sometimes people unconsciously hunch their shoulders when attempting to press their palms together. Until your shoulder flexibility develops, take your palms apart and arms parallel and check if this releases it. If you still feel "bad" shoulder tension, then lower your arms 10 or 20 degrees forward, with attention focused on spreading the shoulder blades well apart.

side angle stretch
parsvakonasana

From the steady base of the legs, you can now reach out with energy to stretch fully the entire side of the body.

1 From Mountain Pose (see page 40), bring the legs into the same position as Warrior II (see page 44). More weight tends to come onto the front leg, so during the pose press into the floor with your back foot to spread your weight evenly between both feet. Stretch your left arm up and out to the side. The right side of the torso will naturally lengthen, so pay particular attention to extending out of your left hip to lengthen the underside of the torso as well.

2 Bring your left elbow to your thigh. Use the elbow to press the knee back so your left inner thigh will lengthen. The kneecap should point in the same direction as your middle toe, not in the direction of your big toe. This elbow pressure aids the twist in the torso so your torso can rotate upward. Stretch your right arm straight up, reaching with your fingers as high as you can. Take a few breaths before proceeding to the full asana. If this is where you stay for today, hold this position for five to ten breaths.

3 For the full pose, bring your left hand to cup the floor near your little toe. With your right arm overhead, turn the palm to the direction you are bending and bring the arm to form a straight line from right foot to right hand. You may need to widen your stance or bend the left knee more to lower your hips. Gaze up to the sky from under your upper arm. Build the time in the pose to 10 breaths. Repeat on the other side.

mighty pose
utkatasana

Don't let your breath harden or become irregular as you hold this strong pose, which strengthens willpower and determination.

1 Stand in Mountain Pose (see page 40) with your big toes and inner heels together. Keeping the heels anchored, deeply bend the knees. Reach out your arms in front of you to press your palms together. Inhale your arms up overhead. If possible, make your elbows straight as you do this. Lift everything up from the hips except the shoulders. Unhunch your shoulders and keep as much distance as you can between your earlobes and upper arms.

2 Gaze upward. Press the pubic bone forward and upward to flatten out the lower back. Draw your abdominal muscles in and up to support this flattening. Work the muscles along the spine strongly to bring it more vertical. Bend the knees to take your hips lower and press the inner thighs together. Stay in position for five breaths.

explore*yoga*

For more of a challenge, to extend this pose, take your thighbones parallel to the floor for five breaths. The trunk will naturally want to lean forward. To deepen the pose, lift the abdomen away from the legs to resist this lean and bring the back more perpendicular to the floor.

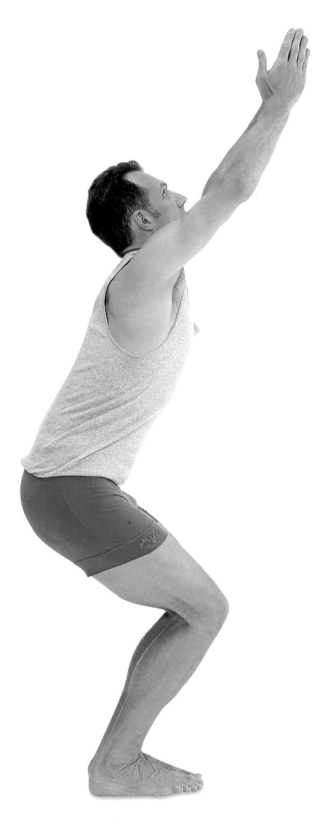

warrior II
virabhadrasana II

As if you were aiming a bow and arrow at your target, maintain a perfect mental focus over your middle finger during this pose. Strong legs give self-reliance and independence and the raised head fosters fearlessness.

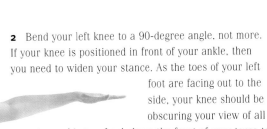

1 From Mountain Pose take the feet wide apart, so that when your arms are stretched out, your ankles will be underneath them. Rotating from the top of the thigh, turn the right leg and foot inward 15 degrees. Turn the left leg and foot out 90 degrees. This tends to alter the position of the hips. Bring your hands onto your hips to help you compare them. If you find your right hip is higher and more forward than the left hip, adjust so that they are in line again.

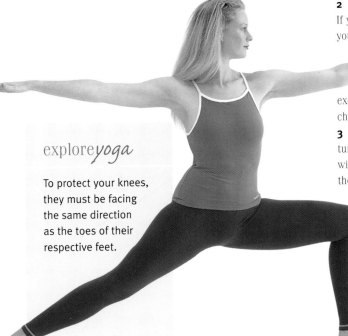

explore*yoga*

To protect your knees, they must be facing the same direction as the toes of their respective feet.

2 Bend your left knee to a 90-degree angle, not more. If your knee is positioned in front of your ankle, then you need to widen your stance. As the toes of your left foot are facing out to the side, your knee should be obscuring your view of all except your big toe. Look down the front of your torso to check that the ribs on both sides are even.

3 Rotate your upper arms outward so that the palms turn out. Then raise your arms until they are parallel with the floor. Finally, rotate just the forearms so that the palms face down to the floor—the creases of your elbows will remain facing upward. Drop your shoulders down. Become aware of two lines of energy radiating from your spine out to your fingertips. Use this feeling to help keep your arms parallel to the floor. Turn your head to gaze at your left index finger. Take ten slow, steady breaths before repeating on the right side.

triangle pose
trikonasana

This pose has five rays of energy: two arms stretching away, two legs stretching out and down, and a fifth line running from the tailbone as it extends toward the crown of the head.

1 From Mountain Pose, jump or step the feet 4–4½ ft (1.2–1.4 m) apart. Turning from the thighs, rotate the right foot inward 15 degrees and turn the left foot out 90 degrees. Level off your hips. If your legs are not working fully, your kneecaps will slump down and inward, so activate your thigh muscles to ensure the kneecaps track over the toes. Take your left hand near your knee. Trikonasana is a strong side stretch so the body needs to be on one plane. Your hipbones, shoulders, and hands should be along the same line as your feet. To open the chest and keep your single-plane alignment, wrap the other arm around the back to wedge the hand by the inner thigh, or else take hold of the back of your trousers. Assist this action by bending the front knee.

2 Draw your left sitting bone down toward your right inner heel so your hips move to the right. As you do this, straighten your left leg and slide the left hand down the leg or possibly to the floor as pictured. If you find your shoulders have come forward of your feet, and your buttocks have moved back, adjust your alignment by bringing your left hand higher up your leg. Roll your right shoulder back and enjoy the openness in the chest for several breaths before eventually releasing your right arm to vertical. Then stretch out well from abdomen to feet, and from shoulders toward each hand. Intensify the line of energy from tailbone to crown of the head by sliding the shoulder blades away from the ears to keep the back of the neck long. Tuck the chin slightly in, turn the head, and gaze at the right thumb. Stay for five to ten breaths, then repeat on the right side.

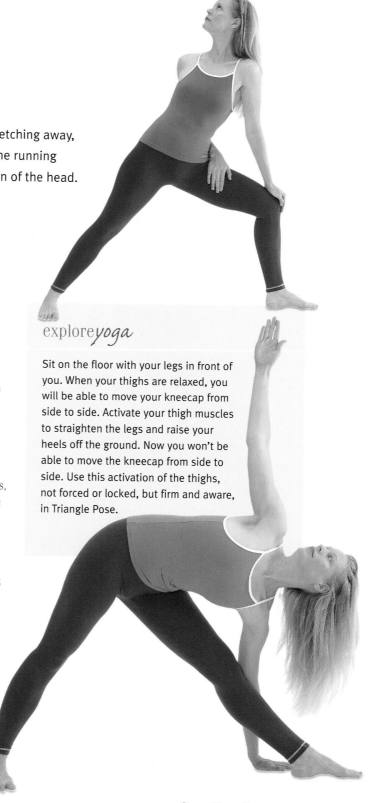

explore yoga

Sit on the floor with your legs in front of you. When your thighs are relaxed, you will be able to move your kneecap from side to side. Activate your thigh muscles to straighten the legs and raise your heels off the ground. Now you won't be able to move the kneecap from side to side. Use this activation of the thighs, not forced or locked, but firm and aware, in Triangle Pose.

wide leg stretch
prasarita padottanasana

In asanas the arms and legs often act as levers to work the spine. But make sure they work with the rest of your body and breath, not forcefully overriding them.

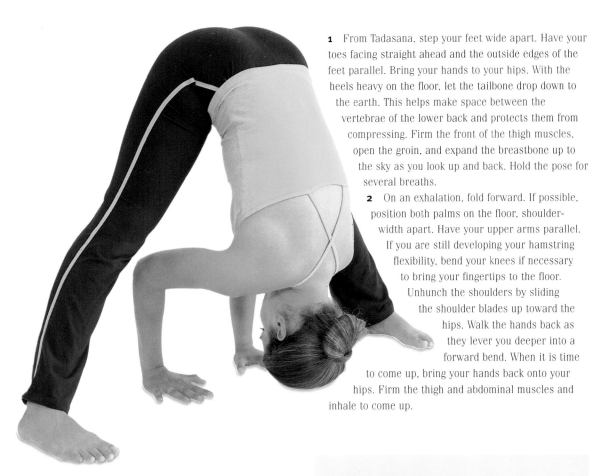

1   From Tadasana, step your feet wide apart. Have your toes facing straight ahead and the outside edges of the feet parallel. Bring your hands to your hips. With the heels heavy on the floor, let the tailbone drop down to the earth. This helps make space between the vertebrae of the lower back and protects them from compressing. Firm the front of the thigh muscles, open the groin, and expand the breastbone up to the sky as you look up and back. Hold the pose for several breaths.

2   On an exhalation, fold forward. If possible, position both palms on the floor, shoulder-width apart. Have your upper arms parallel. If you are still developing your hamstring flexibility, bend your knees if necessary to bring your fingertips to the floor. Unhunch the shoulders by sliding the shoulder blades up toward the hips. Walk the hands back as they lever you deeper into a forward bend. When it is time to come up, bring your hands back onto your hips. Firm the thigh and abdominal muscles and inhale to come up.

explore*yoga*

Interlace your fingers behind your back and take your arms overhead. Firm your front thigh muscles as your thumbs move toward the floor.

intense forward stretch
uttanasana

If you suffer from hypertension, keep the trunk parallel to the floor and place your hands on a chair or table. Begin working through this sequence with Roll Downs (see page 32).

1 To maintain length in the front of the torso, practice using the wall. Stand with your feet apart and about 1 ft (30 cm) away from the wall. Lean your buttocks to the wall so your sitting bones touch it. Hold your elbows and take the arms overhead. Bend the knees and extend the torso up so the top of the breastbone moves away from the pubic bone. With knees strongly bent, reach your torso forward. Stretch as far out with the elbows as possible. Finally fold over your legs and let your upper body hang for ten breaths or more. With each inhalation the torso can lengthen more, and with each exhalation the crease at the top of the thighs can deepen. If you can't work into this position in a relaxed fashion, bend the knees more or walk the feet further away from the wall. Come up on an inhalation.

2 Move away from the wall. Bring your hands on your hips, inhale, lift your breastbone, and look up. Exhale, hinge at the hips to reach forward so the crown of the head

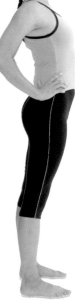
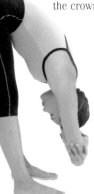

moves in as big an arc as possible. Imagine your hip sockets and pelvis rolling forward over your thighbones, which stay vertical.

3 With your knees bent or straight, grasp your legs or ankles, or loop your big toes with finger and thumb. Increase the stretch by flattening out the back and stretching your sternum forward. Angle your sitting bones toward the sky, lengthen the back of your waist. Tilt your pelvis forward as if aiming to press your navel to your thighs—you will feel the stretch in the back of your thighs intensify.

4 Then exhale and fold forward to hold the pose. If your knees are bent, use each exhalation to work the legs straighter. If your legs are straight, firm the front thigh muscles and bring your hips forward to bring the hip joints directly over your ankles.

5 Check that your face is relaxed. Free the upper lip so your cheeks feel like they are dropping down toward the floor. If you have forgotten to breathe, check whether the pose is too strong for you and ease back until you free the breath.

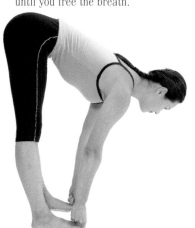
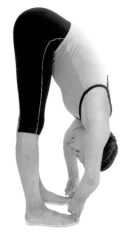

chest to leg extension
parsvottanasana

With your hands in the prayer position behind your back, this strong forward bend will help stretch not only the legs and the chest, but the whole body.

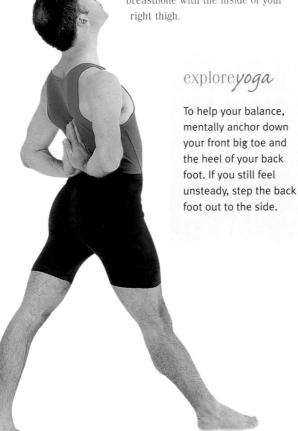

1   From Mountain Pose, take your feet 3–4 ft (1–1.2 m) apart. Turn your left knee and foot deeply inward to 60 degrees, and your right leg and foot out 90 degrees. Your left hip will be further back than your right hip. Bring it forward so both hips are level and you can better line up your breastbone with the inside of your right thigh.

explore*yoga*

To help your balance, mentally anchor down your front big toe and the heel of your back foot. If you still feel unsteady, step the back foot out to the side.

2   To form the prayer position, bring the backs of your hands to your back. Walk your fingers up between the shoulder blades, then roll your shoulders and elbows back as you press the mounds of your thumbs together. An alternative for tighter shoulders is to interlace your hands so your knuckles rest on either side of your spine, or else to grasp your elbows behind your back. As a preparation for folding forward, inhale, lift your chest, and look up.

3   Think forward and out before thinking of the downward movement over your right thigh. Exhale as you reach out of the hips to sweep up, out, forward, and then down. It is easy to bend the knees unknowingly in this pose so keep the thigh muscles activated and press down through the back heel. Stay for five to ten breaths before repeating on the second side.

Alternative
While you develop your flexibility in this pose, practicing using a chair keeps your back straight and your chest open to encourage full breathing.

revolved triangle pose
pavritta trikonasana

This advanced pose combines balance, twisting, and forward bending. In the wide stance poses, the further apart the feet are, the greater the spinal extension, but the more difficult it becomes to balance.

1 Stand with your feet 3–4 ft (1–1.2 m) apart. Turn your left foot and leg well inward to about 60 degrees and turn the right foot out 90 degrees. Bring your left hip forward so that it's level with the right hip. Stretch your left arm up in the air and take several breaths, getting a sense of the full extension all the way from the left ankle to the left hand.

exploreyoga

Looking down to the floor makes it easier to balance while you increase the twist in the trunk. Take several breaths gazing at the floor to allow a deeper rotation. Finally turn the head to look forward and slowly up to the top thumb.

2 On an exhalation, reach the left arm and torso forward and down to bring the left hand to cup the floor by the right little toe. If the hand doesn't reach, place the hand on the seat of a chair or on a stack of books. With both feet and the left hand anchored, stretch the right hip back to help the extension of the spine out of the hips. Rotate the torso well to the right so the navel and heart open up to the sky. Take the right arm straight up into the air and gaze up at your right thumb.

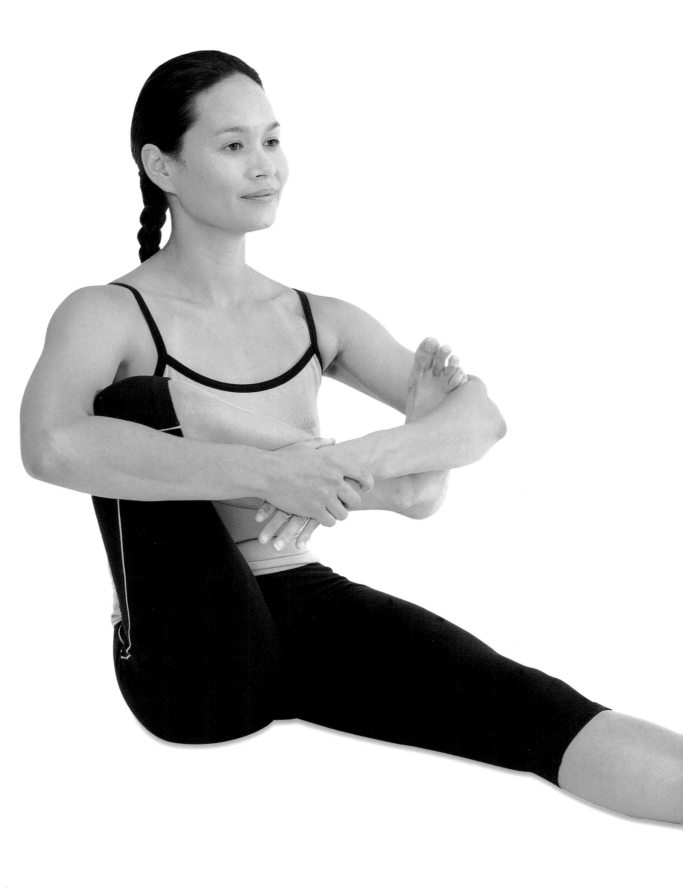

5 ForwardBends

Sometimes in our outward-looking lives, we ignore messages from inside. Folding into ourselves quietens the mind and encourages a meditative mindset. Forward bends foster the ability to listen to our intuitive self, to our heart.

Gravity often helps us fold forward; we can go deeper into the pose by yielding rather than forcing. From the seated position, we don't even have to be concerned with balancing, and can take energy and support from the earth. The forward bends are a little like the fetal position and have nurturing qualities for when we need to feel protected.

As you fold in half from your hips, your head comes closer to your feet. The two extremes of the body come together and help you find your center. Life is full of dualities. Rather than operating from one end of the spectrum, you can find a better balance; moderation and the middle path in our world view and way of living.

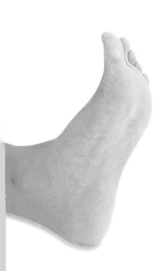

about *alignment*

It's worthwhile investing some time to discover how to get the most benefit out of forward bends.

1 Sit erect in your chair and place your hands on your waist. Lower your chin to your chest, then bring your head down toward your thighs. You will feel the stretch mostly along the sides of the spine. Observe how your shoulders hunch and your back rounds. You might also notice that it's difficult to take deep breaths.

2 Now sit up straight once again and lower your hands from your waist to your hips. Inhale, expand the chest, lengthen your spine up, and gaze forward. As you exhale, fold forward, leading with the chest. With this movement you hinge from the hips. Compared with the last exercise, the spine is kept relatively straight (which protects the intervertebral discs) and you will feel the stretch more in the hips and backs of the thighs than in the spine. This is the movement required by the yoga forward bends. Practice these two variations a couple more times so you are clear in your mind about the difference. Imprint the memory of this second exercise in your body so you can bring it alive during every yoga forward bend you will encounter in the future.

> DON'T OVERDO THE FORWARD BENDS IF YOU SUFFER FROM SEVERE DEPRESSION. FOCUS ON BACKBENDS INSTEAD. THOSE SUFFERING HYPERTENSION DO BEST TO KEEP THEIR HEAD ABOVE THEIR HEART. FORWARD BENDS MAINTAIN INTEGRITY OF THE SPINE, BUT PROCEED CAUTIOUSLY IF YOU HAVE BACK PAIN. IF A WEAKNESS EXISTS OR IF YOU ARE RECOVERING FROM AN INJURY, IT IS ALWAYS BEST TO BUILD YOUR PRACTICE IN A SLOW AND STEADY WAY. IF YOU SUFFER FROM DISC PROBLEMS, THAT SECTION OF THE SPINE NEEDS TO BE KEPT CONCAVE AND SHOULD NOT BE BENT FORWARD UNTIL IT IS READY.

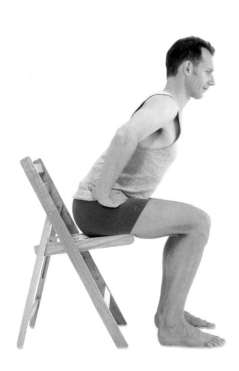

3 It helps if we understand where we place our seat when sitting erect. The two sitting bones (ischial tuberosities) act as little anchors to the earth. As you sit on the floor, reach under your buttocks and move your buttock flesh away, in a direction 45 degrees back and out to the side, to help your sitting bones to make contact with the ground.

4 If you have a lack of flexibility in the hamstrings, you will tend to sit on the back edge of your sitting bones. The pelvis will be tilted backward, as the tight hamstrings pull around the corner on the lower back and flatten the normal lumbar curve. Your stomach muscles have to work hard to keep you upright, so sitting in this position won't be comfortable. It also creates a tendency to concave the chest. A forward bend born from this position will inevitably be a forward bend from the waist, instead of the hips. Apart from closing the chest to deep breathing, by pressuring the fronts of the intervertebral discs, the spine will not maintain a healthy alignment. The ideal starting position will be sitting right on the center of the sitting bones so that as you fold your body forward, you will roll forward to perch more on the front edge of your sitting bones.

5 While sitting on the floor, touch your lower back. If your lower back still flattens or rounds out instead of keeping its usual inward curve, then your pelvis will be tilting backward. As you need to move from sitting on the back edge of the sitting bones to being on their center, modify your starting position. Lift your seat with folded blankets, and/or bend your knees. Use one or both of these adjustments in your forward bends for as many months as it takes for your body to loosen.

6 It is better to do a smaller-looking forward bend with correct alignment than a seemingly deeper forward bend, which at worst may be injurious and at best doesn't really help release the areas that are chronically tight. Keep the length in the spine by extending the tailbone and crown of the head away from each other. As you fold forward, stretch your tailbone back and away from the crown of the head. Moving the sitting bones back increases the stretch in the hamstrings.

7 As you fold forward, visualize your thighbones staying still. It is actually the sockets of the hip joints that can rotate around the heads of the thighbones to tilt the pelvis forward. When you can achieve this, the concavity in the lumbar spine will remain for the first part of the forward bend. Test this by placing your hand on your lower back to feel if you have the same curve during the first part of the forward bend. Toward the end of your stretch forward, you will feel the lumbar spine begin to curve outward.

8 Let go of your desire to reach your forehead to your knees. Instead, first aim the navel to the thighs. As you hinge more at the hips, your chest will come closer to your knees, and only after this will the nose come toward the shins.

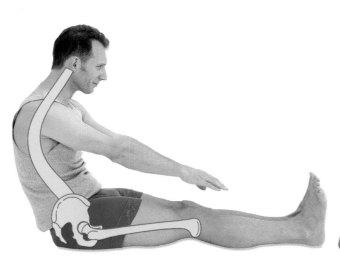 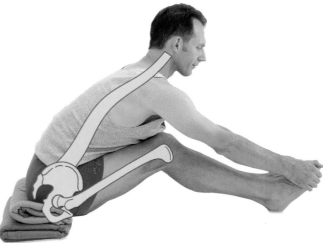

staff pose
dandasana

The dandasana pose is the base from which we fold forward into many of the forward bends. Because this position is outwardly simpler and easier to master than many others, it provides a good opportunity to take your attention inward.

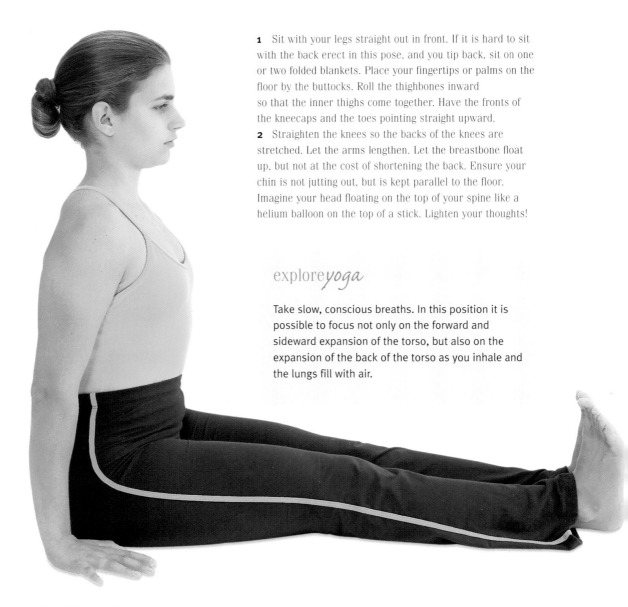

1 Sit with your legs straight out in front. If it is hard to sit with the back erect in this pose, and you tip back, sit on one or two folded blankets. Place your fingertips or palms on the floor by the buttocks. Roll the thighbones inward so that the inner thighs come together. Have the fronts of the kneecaps and the toes pointing straight upward.

2 Straighten the knees so the backs of the knees are stretched. Let the arms lengthen. Let the breastbone float up, but not at the cost of shortening the back. Ensure your chin is not jutting out, but is kept parallel to the floor. Imagine your head floating on the top of your spine like a helium balloon on the top of a stick. Lighten your thoughts!

explore*yoga*

Take slow, conscious breaths. In this position it is possible to focus not only on the forward and sideward expansion of the torso, but also on the expansion of the back of the torso as you inhale and the lungs fill with air.

hero pose
virasana

Although children sit like this quite naturally, older, stiffer bodies can find this pose uncomfortable. Use props as necessary while you regain your flexibility.

1 Kneel on the floor with your knees together and feet wide apart. As you sit down between your feet, use your fingers to "iron" your calf muscles out to the sides and down toward the heels.

2 Place your hands on the soles of your upturned feet. Lift up from your pubic bone to the notch of the throat. Lift up on the back of the body too, from the tailbone to the crown of the head.

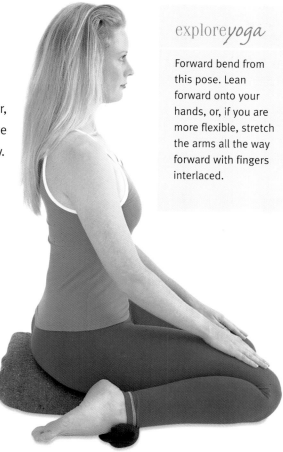

explore*yoga*

Forward bend from this pose. Lean forward onto your hands, or, if you are more flexible, stretch the arms all the way forward with fingers interlaced.

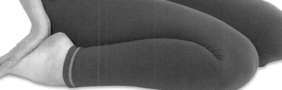

3 If your buttocks don't come down to the floor, then create as much height as you need to be comfortable but still with a degree of challenge. Use a pillow, folded blankets, or an old telephone book as a prop; each time you practice, tear out a few pages or fold the blanket less thickly so that, over time, you are able to sit comfortably on the floor.

4 If you experience knee pain, place a canvas belt or thin, folded scarf deeply in the crease of the knees as they bend.

5 If this position gives pain on the tops of the feet, place some cushioning underneath the fronts of the ankles to make it more comfortable.

three-limbed forward bend
trianga mukhaikapada paschimottanasana

If forward-bending Hero Pose is too much of a challenge for now, warm yourself up by practicing one leg at a time.

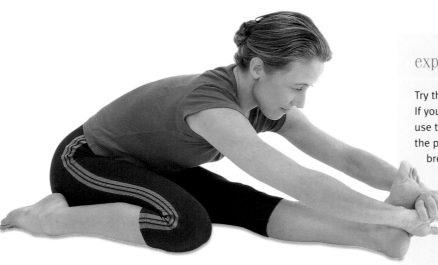

explore*yoga*

Try this way of working in some poses. If you will hold a pose for ten breaths, use the first five to adjust and deepen the posture. For the remaining five breaths, remain steady at a still point. At this point you still the fluctuations of the body, and are moving neither from nor toward any point. Be receptive to your observations.

1 From Dandasana (see page 54), bend your right leg back to bring the foot to the floor next to the buttocks. As in Virasana (see page 55), "iron" your calf flesh out to the right. As you will tend to tilt to the left, maintain balance by mentally letting your right sitting bone be heavy.

2 Sometimes it is useful to use a flowing movement to ease yourself into a pose. On an inhalation, reach your arms up to the sky and then fold forward as you exhale. On the next inhalation, reach the arms out and up once more, and flow forward as you exhale. After five cycles, hold the forward bend for five to ten long breaths. Then repeat on the other side.

Alternative

To align the spine and better balance the hips, place a support under one buttock.

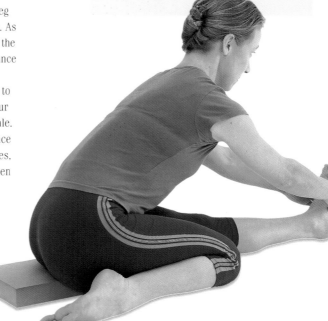

head beyond the knee pose
janu sirsasana

As this pose stretches out the lower back, it is wonderful after backbends and inversions.

1   From Dandasana (see page 54), bend your right leg out to the side so the sole of the foot comes close to, but not actually touching, the left inner thigh. Keep your left leg straight by opening the back of the knee to the floor.

2   Stretch your left heel away so the knee and toes point straight up. Tilt the pelvis forward so you are sitting on the front side of the sitting bones. Before you think about going forward, it's useful to sit erect and breathe yourself taller for a short while. When you are ready, inhale your arms overhead.

3   Exhale as you extend forward to grasp your calf, ankle, or foot. Inhale, lift your chest, and look up. Exhale, bend your elbows to the side, and fold forward maintaining a flat back and open chest. Hold five to ten breaths before repeating the other side.

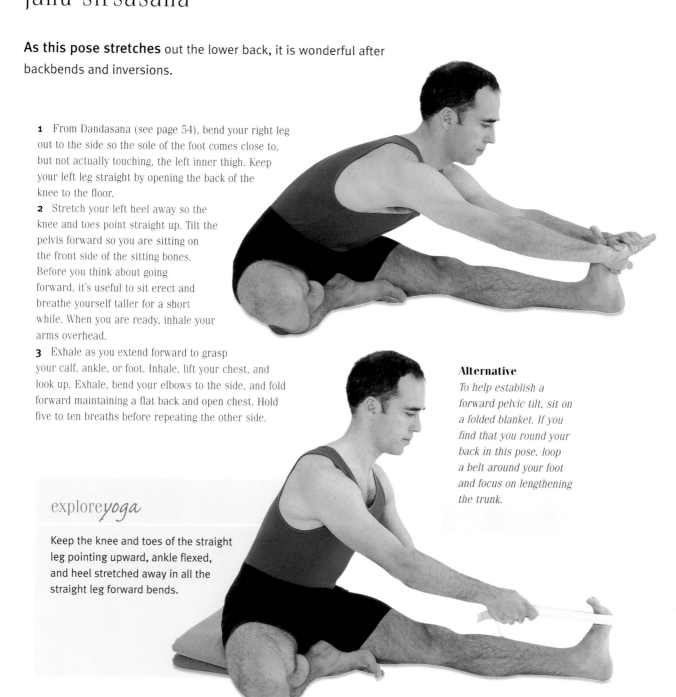

Alternative
To help establish a forward pelvic tilt, sit on a folded blanket. If you find that you round your back in this pose, loop a belt around your foot and focus on lengthening the trunk.

explore*yoga*

Keep the knee and toes of the straight leg pointing upward, ankle flexed, and heel stretched away in all the straight leg forward bends.

bound half lotus forward fold
ardha baddha padma paschimottanasana

Due to the position of the arms in this hip-opening stretch, it is difficult to "cheat" by rounding the shoulders. Warming up the hip will help prevent knee problems and assist the movement of the knee toward the earth.

1 Warm up the hip by cradling your right leg. If cradling is difficult, then hold the knee and foot in both hands and push them slightly together. Slowly move the leg back and forth as you would rock a baby. Keep your right foot flexed as you slowly move the knee beyond the armpit. If you find this movement easy, then lift the right foot up higher.

2 Take the bent leg to the floor and out to the side. Hold the top of the foot, and slide it onto the other thigh until the ankle is resting on the thigh—if you only bring the top of the foot to the thigh, the ligaments of the outside of the foot risk being overstretched. Reach around with your right hand and take hold of the foot.

3 Stretch forward and take your right hand to the right foot, ankle, or shin. Release your left knee down to the floor. Hold for five to ten breaths. Repeat from the beginning on the other side.

Alternative
If you can't reach, loop a belt around your shin and hold both ends with your left hand.

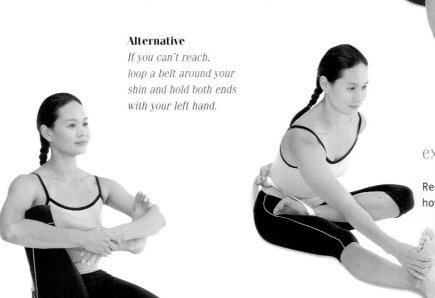

explore*yoga*

Remind yourself that it is irrelevant how far you look like you go in a pose. The important thing is to reach the point where you can learn and change. Measure your posture not by how flexible you are, but by how steady your breath is.

stretch on the west side of the body
paschimottanasana

Traditionally yoga asana practice is done facing north or east. In this pose, as you fold toward the east, you stretch the side of the body facing west.

1 Sit tall in Dandasana (see page 54) and wriggle forward so you come onto the front edge of your sitting bones. If your hamstrings are tight and you feel your torso leaning backward, instead of being vertical, then sit on folded blankets and/or bend your knees up a little.

2 To avoid the undesirable habit of rounding the back, first experiment with the position of your arms. Bring your hands into the prayer pose behind the back (as in Parsvottanasana on page 48). If you find this too difficult, cup both elbows behind your back.

3 On an exhalation, fold forward, tilting the pelvis forward and using your abdominal muscles. The position of the arms means your chest is kept open.

4 Stay and breathe. You should feel your palms spread apart as the back of the trunk expands with each inhalation. If you can't access this movement, ease off on the intensity until you are able to free up the back for the breath. Imprint this feeling of the straight back and open chest on your body's memory, so that you can repeat it during the next stage.

5 Now practice the classic Paschimottanasana. Sit in Dandasana. Keep your knees and toes pointing to the sky. Lengthen from the tailbone to the crown of the head. After several breaths "growing" the spine, inhale and raise the arms overhead, then exhale the arms and torso forward. Remember the feeling from the first exercise—keep the chest open and the breath free. Depending on your flexibility, hold one wrist around the feet, hook your toes, grasp the sides of your feet or ankles, or loop a belt around the balls of the feet. Take long, slow breaths for ten to fifteen rounds.

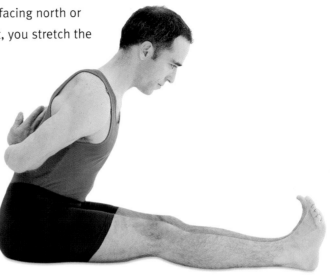

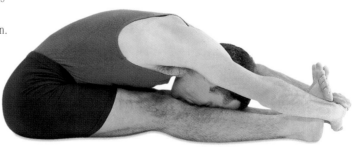

explore*yoga*

Experiment with different arm positions in this pose. Try bending forward with the arms in the Cow Face Pose (see page 64), interlacing your fingers at the back of the neck, or with your fingers interlaced behind your back and arms lifting up.

seated wide angle pose sequence
upavista konasana

Have patience as you hold this pose. Wait for the body to let you in.

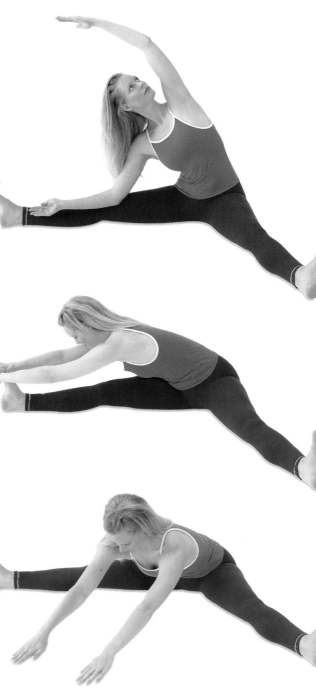

1 Sit with your legs out to the sides at about a 90-degree angle. In this pose it is easy to let the kneecaps roll backward or forward so check that your kneecaps and toes point straight up. Place your right hand, palm up, on your right thigh. Inhale and raise your left arm up, then curve over to the right so the sides of your body curve out like a rainbow. Keep your left shoulder on the same plane as your right, not in front of it. "Puff" out the left side ribs and draw the right side ribs into the body. Imagine the spaces between the left sides of each vertebra stretching apart. Slide your right hand down your leg. Hold for at least five breaths.

2 Now twist your torso toward the floor as you lower your left shoulder and arm. Bring the left hand near the right to stretch over your right leg. Turn the toes back and extend through the heels. Anchor down through the left sitting bone. Hold for five to ten breaths.

3 Now you have arrived at Upavista Konasana. Walk the hands in a wide arc toward the center. Ease back a little so you can tune into the sensation of the trunk lifting out of the hips. Slide the hands forward as you release in stages over about a minute.

4 When you have completed this sequence on both sides of the body, support under your knees with your hands as you bring your legs together for Dandasana.

> **!** YOU SHOULD NOT EXPERIENCE INNER KNEE PAIN IN THIS POSE. IF YOU DO, MAKE SURE YOU ARE WORKING THE LEGS BY STRETCHING OUT THROUGH THE HEELS, AND FIRMING THE THIGH MUSCLES TO THE BONE. NARROW THE DISTANCE BETWEEN THE LEGS AND EASE OFF ON THE STRETCH.

cobbler's pose
baddha konasana

Translated from Sanskrit as Bound Angle Pose, this position is also called Cobbler's Pose because it is the position in which shoemakers in India sit to work.

1 Raise your seat with a support like a cushion and bring the soles of your feet together. Draw your heels up close toward you. Use the pressure of your hands on the floor behind you to tilt the pelvis forward. As you do so, let the breastbone float up. These two movements will begin the opening along the inner thighs and groin. With the support of your hands behind you, move the knees away from each other, back and down to the floor. If your hips are tight, this may be as far as you go in this pose for today.

2 If your pelvis tips forward easily, you can dispense with the cushion before bending your elbows into the calves and binding the feet with your hands. Inhale and create the sensation of the torso lifting out of the pelvis. Exhale and deepen the fold. On each inhalation, lengthen right up from pubic bone to throat; each exhalation is an opportunity to move out and down. Rather than butterflying the knees up and down, work with the breath to soften the tight areas. Breathe evenly and repeat for five to ten rounds.

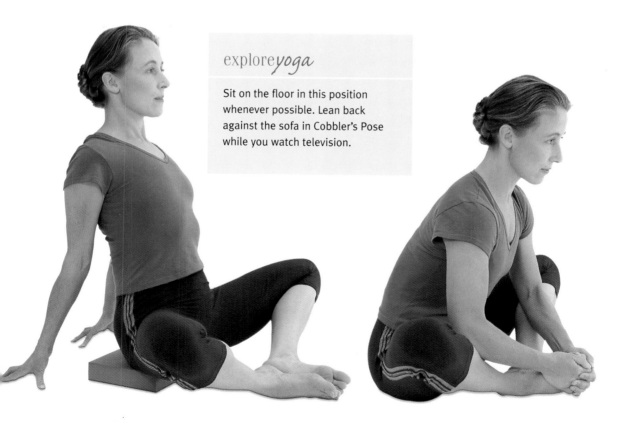

explore*yoga*

Sit on the floor in this position whenever possible. Lean back against the sofa in Cobbler's Pose while you watch television.

reclining big toe pose

reclining big toe pose

This pose keeps the back stable and helps prevent it from overstretching by moving the stretch more into the hamstrings. For those who are recovering from a herniated disc, this pose is a safe forward bend to practice on the road to recovery.

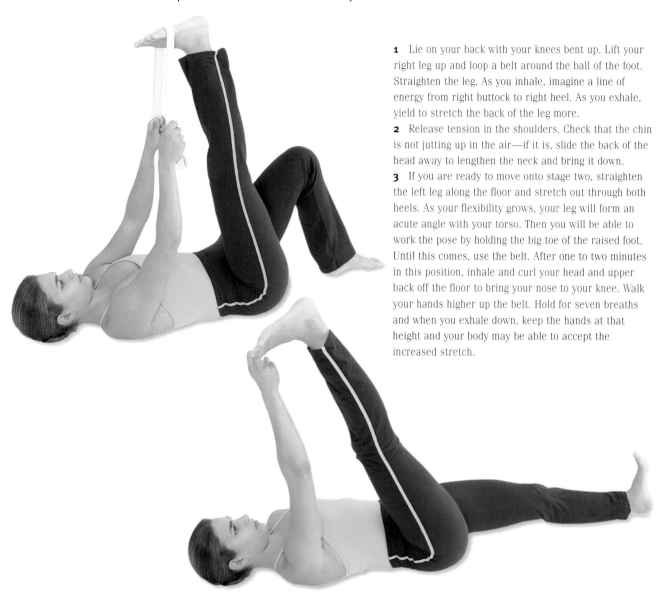

1 Lie on your back with your knees bent up. Lift your right leg up and loop a belt around the ball of the foot. Straighten the leg. As you inhale, imagine a line of energy from right buttock to right heel. As you exhale, yield to stretch the back of the leg more.

2 Release tension in the shoulders. Check that the chin is not jutting up in the air—if it is, slide the back of the head away to lengthen the neck and bring it down.

3 If you are ready to move onto stage two, straighten the left leg along the floor and stretch out through both heels. As your flexibility grows, your leg will form an acute angle with your torso. Then you will be able to work the pose by holding the big toe of the raised foot. Until this comes, use the belt. After one to two minutes in this position, inhale and curl your head and upper back off the floor to bring your nose to your knee. Walk your hands higher up the belt. Hold for seven breaths and when you exhale down, keep the hands at that height and your body may be able to accept the increased stretch.

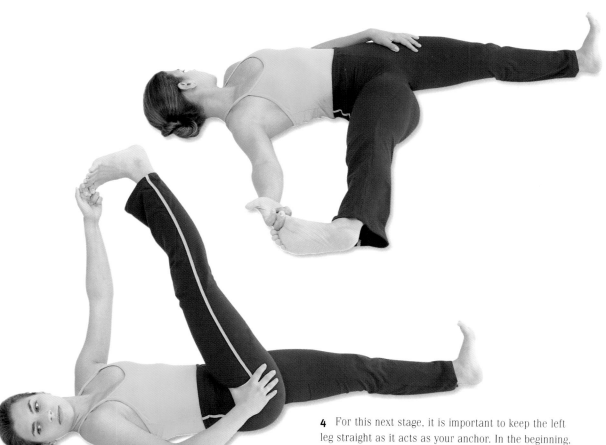

exploreyoga

Before you do this hip-releasing sequence, lie flat and look at your feet. Your toes will be turned out— measure how much the toes of each foot are turned out, checking the difference between sides. This sequence releases the hips. Visually measure it again after each side.

4 For this next stage, it is important to keep the left leg straight as it acts as your anchor. In the beginning, use your left hand to press down on the top of your left thigh. Holding the belt or side of your foot, take your right leg out to the side. Although you may not get that high this practice, aim to take your toes to the floor at shoulder level. Do this movement slowly so you don't lose the grounding force of the left upper thigh and left heel. If you start to tip, come back up and press both sides of the sacrum down to the floor before lowering down again. Hold for five to ten breaths.

5 Come back to center and hold your big toe, or both ends of the belt, in your left hand. Turn your toes inward and anchor down the sacrum on the right side. It helps to press down with your thumb at the root of the thigh. Take the leg over to the left and hold for five to ten breaths. Come back to stretching through the center before lowering the leg down to repeat from the beginning on the other side.

cow face pose
gomukhasana

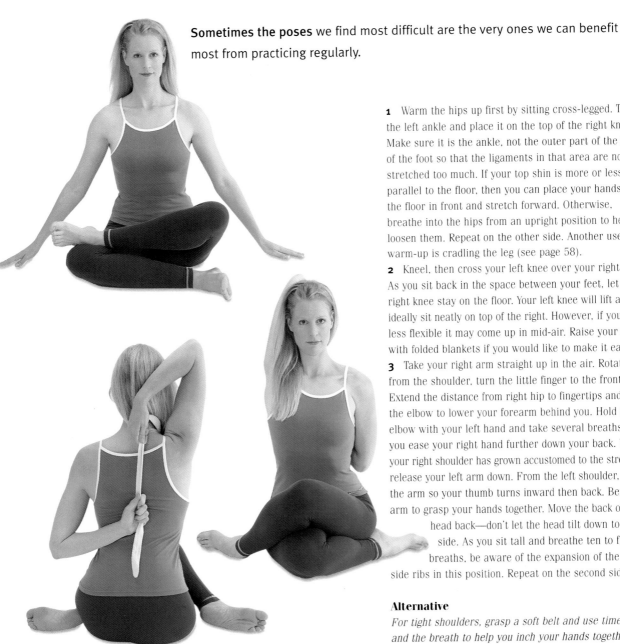

Sometimes the poses we find most difficult are the very ones we can benefit most from practicing regularly.

1 Warm the hips up first by sitting cross-legged. Take the left ankle and place it on the top of the right knee. Make sure it is the ankle, not the outer part of the top of the foot so that the ligaments in that area are not stretched too much. If your top shin is more or less parallel to the floor, then you can place your hands on the floor in front and stretch forward. Otherwise, breathe into the hips from an upright position to help loosen them. Repeat on the other side. Another useful warm-up is cradling the leg (see page 58).

2 Kneel, then cross your left knee over your right knee. As you sit back in the space between your feet, let your right knee stay on the floor. Your left knee will lift and ideally sit neatly on top of the right. However, if you are less flexible it may come up in mid-air. Raise your seat with folded blankets if you would like to make it easier.

3 Take your right arm straight up in the air. Rotating from the shoulder, turn the little finger to the front. Extend the distance from right hip to fingertips and bend the elbow to lower your forearm behind you. Hold the elbow with your left hand and take several breaths as you ease your right hand further down your back. When your right shoulder has grown accustomed to the stretch, release your left arm down. From the left shoulder, rotate the arm so your thumb turns inward then back. Bend the arm to grasp your hands together. Move the back of the head back—don't let the head tilt down to one side. As you sit tall and breathe ten to fifteen breaths, be aware of the expansion of the right side ribs in this position. Repeat on the second side.

Alternative

For tight shoulders, grasp a soft belt and use time and the breath to help you inch your hands together.

after *forward folding*

These stretches act as counter poses after some intense forward bending.

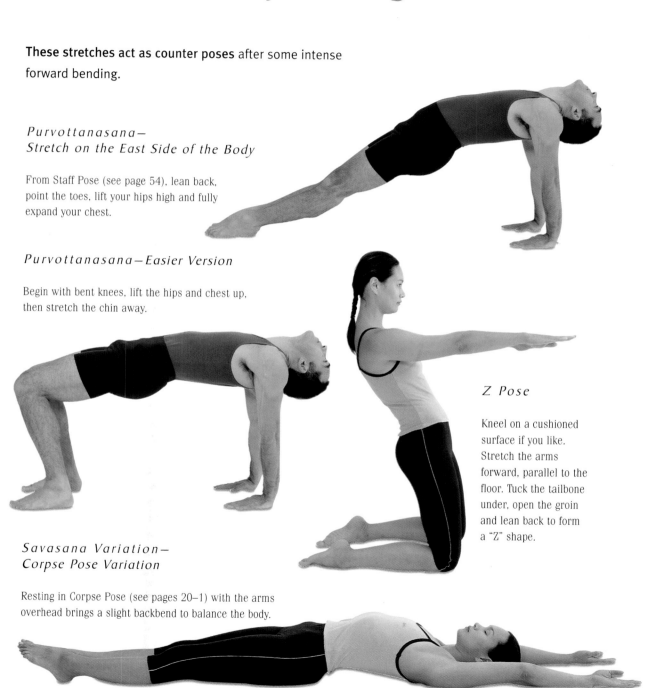

Purvottanasana— Stretch on the East Side of the Body

From Staff Pose (see page 54), lean back, point the toes, lift your hips high and fully expand your chest.

Purvottanasana—Easier Version

Begin with bent knees, lift the hips and chest up, then stretch the chin away.

Z Pose

Kneel on a cushioned surface if you like. Stretch the arms forward, parallel to the floor. Tuck the tailbone under, open the groin and lean back to form a "Z" shape.

Savasana Variation— Corpse Pose Variation

Resting in Corpse Pose (see pages 20–1) with the arms overhead brings a slight backbend to balance the body.

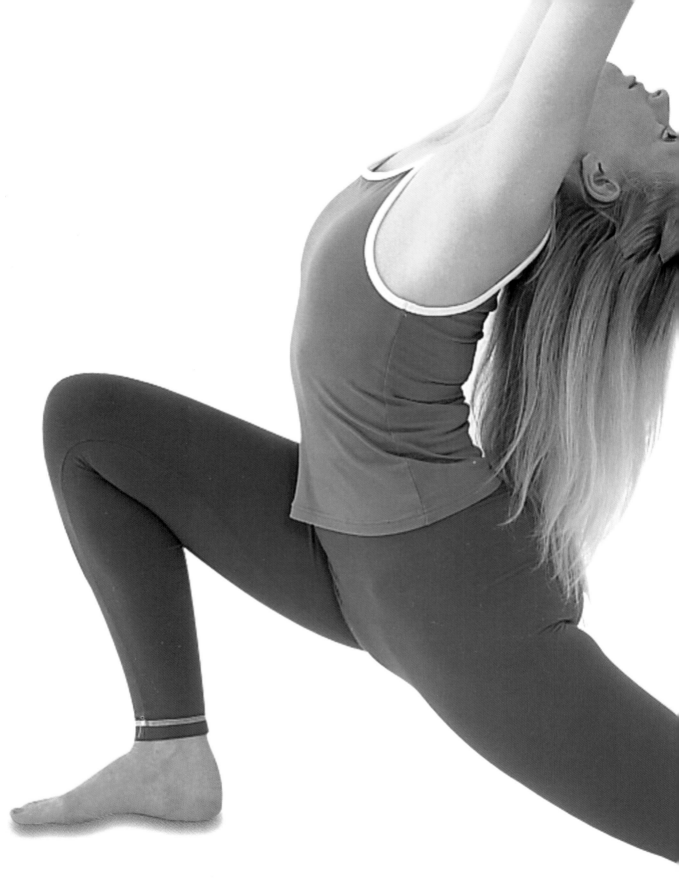

6   Backbends

Like the forward bends, the backbends help keep the spine supple and well aligned to promote good functioning of the nerves that innervate the rest of the body. If you think of what you do every day, you will notice many of your activities involve bending forward. Sitting at a desk to work, at a table to eat, or when driving, even doing housework or gardening, all tend to shorten the front of the body. The common habit of looking at the ground while walking can also put a stoop into otherwise good posture. Backbends realign the spine, counteract rounded shoulders, and help us move with poise and grace.

Always warm up with some standing postures before beginning backbends. To really feel your backbends develop, repeat the pose three times. The body does tend to feel the effects of holding backbends, so follow with some of the counter poses on page 77.

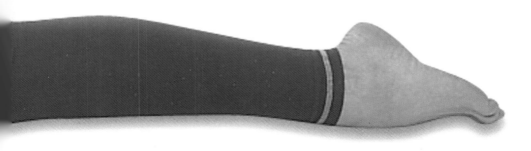

about alignment

Stretch the legs and trunk and open the shoulders before backbending. Warm up the body with these exercises and your backbending will come more easily.

Neck Extension

Elongating the neck teaches you how to extend it in backbends without compressing the cervical spine.

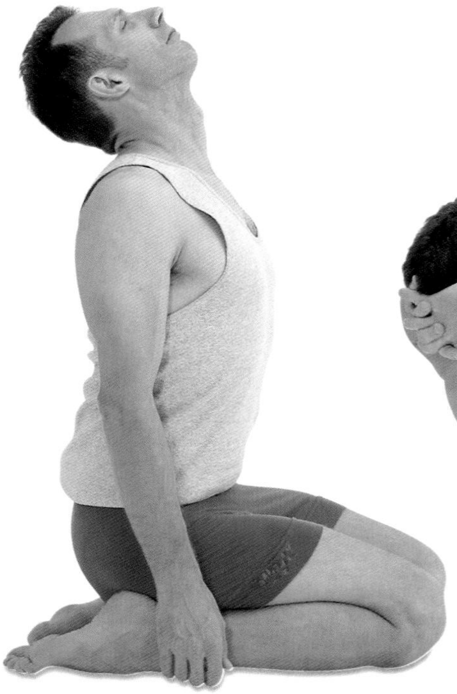

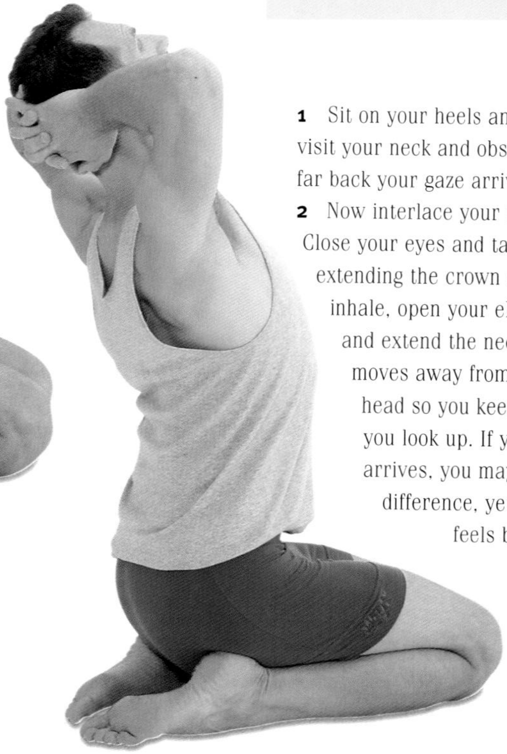

explore*yoga*

If possible, from the Reclining Hero pose pictured opposite, come all the way down to lie on your back. To deepen the backbend, cup an elbow in each palm and take your arms overhead, bringing the elbows to touch the floor. Rest for up to several minutes, then release in Child Pose (see page 19).

1 Sit on your heels and drop your head back. Mentally visit your neck and observe how that feels. Notice how far back your gaze arrives as the head drops back.
2 Now interlace your fingers at the base of your skull. Close your eyes and take a moment to "grow" the neck, extending the crown of the head skyward. As you inhale, open your elbows out to the sides and back, and extend the neck so the back of your head moves away from your shoulders. Cradle your head so you keep the back of the neck long as you look up. If you measure where your gaze arrives, you may notice that there is not a large difference, yet more likely that this option feels better on your neck than the previous one. This feeling of the neck staying long is what you are aiming for in backbends like the Cobra and Locust Poses.

Shoulder Extension

These shoulder exercises give more lift with "longer" released arms.

1 Stand side-on to the wall, at a distance of about 10 in (25 cm). The more flexible you are, the closer you will get to the wall. Stretch the arm closest to the wall as high up as you can reach, touching your palm to wall. Take several slow breaths, feeling like you are hanging down from the raised hand. Now take it back 45 degrees (pictured) for another ten or so breaths. Finally, take it further behind, to be, if possible, parallel to the floor. Lean your chest forward and breathe. After doing one side, if you relax your arms and then swing them together to join the palms you might find the worked arm "longer" than the other. Repeat on the other side.

2 Bring your elbows to the padded edge of a table so they are shoulder-width apart. Step back so your ankles are under your hips and you form a table shape. Bring your palms together and lower the head, if possible, so the neck is in line with the spine. You will feel a stretch in the shoulders. This is table prayer pose. As you hold the position, let the side ribs soften down. After ten breaths here, slowly lower your hands between your shoulder blades so your fingers point toward your tailbone. Move slowly between these two positions a few times. To come up, walk in, lift your head, and scoop up.

> **!** IF YOU SUFFER FROM HEART TROUBLE OR HYPERTENSION YOU SHOULD WORK WITH AN EXPERIENCED TEACHER. AVOID STRONG BACKBENDS DURING MENSTRUATION, PREGNANCY, AFTER RECENT SURGERY, FOR EIGHT WEEKS AFTER GIVING BIRTH OR IF YOU SUFFER FROM A HERNIATED DISC, LUMBAR INJURY, OR A PEPTIC OR DUODENAL HERNIA. IF YOU DISCOVER ANY WEAKNESS OF OR DISCOMFORT IN THE BACK, BUILD UP YOUR PRACTICE SLOWLY.

Reclining Hero Pose— Supta Virasana

The ileopsoas is a deep muscle running from the inner thighbone to the lumbar vertebrae. When this muscle is tight or contracted, it pulls us into a forward bend. A released ileopsoas muscle is essential for healthy backbending. Begin in Hero Pose (see page 55). Lean back on your elbows, then come up a little so you can lift your pubic bone up as you stretch your tailbone away. Breathe here for a while. Maintaining the tilt of the pelvis, keep your floating ribs from jutting out as you lower your buttocks to the floor. Gaze straight ahead or take the head back and stretch the chin away. If this stretch is too strong on the thighs, practice the lunge outlined in the first part of Crescent Moon Pose (see page 70), and Warrior I (see page 41).

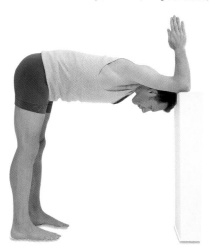

crescent moon pose

anjaneyasana

The ileopsoas-lengthening lunge part of this pose is a good warm-up for all the other backbends. There are two directions of movement of energy in this pose. The movement from the back of the waist down extends out through the back foot and allows the hips to descend. The upward stretch beginning at the waist radiates energy upwards.

1 Kneel on a cushioned surface and step your left leg forward. Cup the floor with your fingertips and bring the hips forward to lunge. Ground through the back knee as you allow time and the breath to further open the left groin and descend the hips. Give the muscles time to relax in this pose. When you have connected to the grounding force of gravity and the hips have got the message to drop, lower the chest down slightly, lengthen forward with the breast bone, press the fingertips to the floor, and lift up to increase the bend in the back. Then practice on the other side.

2 Return to lunge on the first side. When you have followed the same steps, bring your hands to your front knee. Then, reach the arms forward and cross the fingers for strength. Lift the upper body up to the sky. Imagine that someone is gently pulling you by your wrists up out of your hips. At the same time, release the hips so that they sink more to the floor. If the pressure of your back knee against the floor is uncomfortable, press down more through the top of the back foot. If you are comfortable and feel you have a good lifting sensation, you can proceed to the next step.

3 Lengthen the spine further, then lift the breastbone up, curve the back backward, and bring the shoulders and arms back. Drop the head back and stretch the chin away. Inhale to come out of the pose and repeat with the right leg forward.

locust pose
salabhasana

This pose is very strengthening for the back. Due to the pressure on the abdomen it improves digestive function.

1 Lie face down with your forehead on the floor and your arms out in front of you. Have your arms and legs slightly apart. Slightly tilt your pelvis by pressuring your pubic bone to the floor. When you do this, you can reach your toes back further and the back of the waist lengthens.

2 Stretch your right arm and left leg away from each other. Tune into the opposite forces extending from your center of gravity below the navel to your toes and fingertips. Raise your head and lift up your right arm and left leg, continually stretching them away. Hold for several breaths before repeating on the opposite side.

3 After this warm-up, you are ready for Salabhasana. Bring your feet together and your arms by your sides. With your forehead on the floor, tuck your toes under, stretch your heels away and lift up your knees. Firm your thighs and keep both legs straight.

4 After several breaths, flick your toes away and lift your legs up in the air. Keep your inner ankles together. Re-anchor well through the pubic bone. Then lift your arms, head and chest up. Reach back with your fingers toward your toes to deepen the pose. Hold for five to ten breaths. Repeat three times.

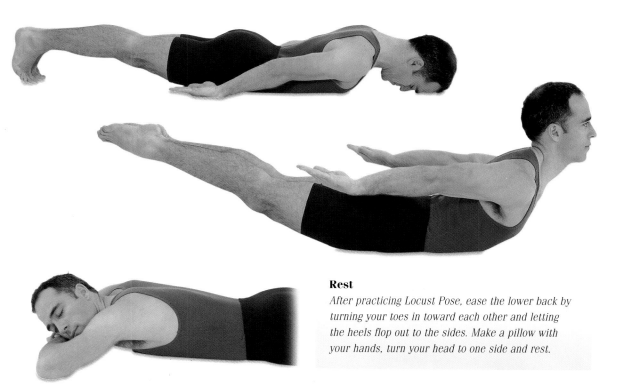

Rest
After practicing Locust Pose, ease the lower back by turning your toes in toward each other and letting the heels flop out to the sides. Make a pillow with your hands, turn your head to one side and rest.

cobra pose
bhujangasana

Though it might look simple, this pose requires determination and strength. Each time you take an inhalation, your abdominal organs benefit from the massage as your abdomen expands into the floor.

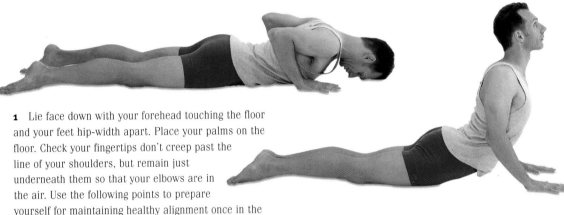

1 Lie face down with your forehead touching the floor and your feet hip-width apart. Place your palms on the floor. Check your fingertips don't creep past the line of your shoulders, but remain just underneath them so that your elbows are in the air. Use the following points to prepare yourself for maintaining healthy alignment once in the pose. Slide your shoulder blades down away from your ears towards your hips. Squeeze your elbows towards each other. Move your tailbone towards your feet and stretch your toes away to elongate the back.

2 Raise your hands 1 in (2.5 cm) off the floor, then lift your head, shoulders, and chest. Mentally check in with the muscles of your back to feel which ones are working to hold you in place. Bring your hands back to the floor. Lengthen your tailbone and breastbone in opposite directions and then pressurize your palms on the floor. Don't let this pose depend entirely on the strength of your arms. Use your arms to assist, but not override the work in the back. Most people will have their hips on the floor with arms well bent. Very flexible people may have straight arms. Hold for five to ten breaths. After three repetitions, use Child Pose (see page 19) or Downward-Facing Dog (see page 96) to release your back.

explore*yoga*

From the shoulders down, the outer body encasing this central core moves down towards your toes. Visualize the inner body elongating with each breath. Your sternum lifts up like the "chest" of the cobra as you rise up to face and overcome any obstruction you face.

Incorrect

Maintain the integrity of the pose. Don't hunch the shoulders or bend the elbows out to the side. Spread the stretch evenly through the spine and back of the neck rather than collapsing at the neck.

camel pose
ustrasana

Forming the camel's hump strongly stretches the thighs, opens the groin, and lifts the heart. The fifth chakra at the throat is activated in this posture with the head tilted back and the chin stretched away.

1 Kneel (on a cushioned surface if you prefer) with your knees hip-width apart. Place your right hand on your lower back and stretch the other one straight up in the air. Push your hips forward and lift up the breastbone. Use the raised arm to give you a lift as you extend back. Keep the head and neck in line with the upper arm and breathe freely. Repeat on side two before sitting down on the heels.

2 While kneeling, tuck your toes under. This time, lift up well through the top arm and bring the other arm down so your fingers hold the heel. Don't twist the body. Keep both hips and front ribs facing forward. After five breaths, repeat on the other side. You are now warmed up for the full Ustrasana.

3 From kneeling, take both hands to the small of your back and massage it a little. The energy moves down from the back of the waist to ground through the knees. Remember the feeling of lift that the raised arms gave to the first two exercises. Maintain the lift through the spine from the back of the waist upward to open the chest. Take the hands one by one to the heels. Then use them as your anchor to open the groin and stretch the hips forward, aiming to have the thighbones vertical. Continue to lift the breastbone to the sky as you roll your shoulders back. Finally, take your head back. When it is time to come up, pressure your feet on the floor, inhale, and come up. After three repetitions, release the back by using Child Pose (see page 19).

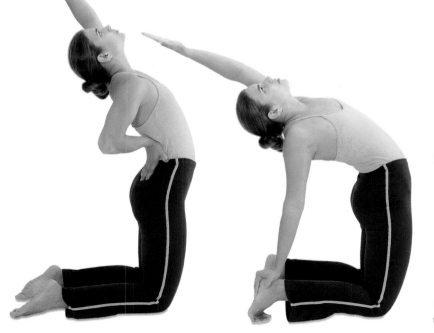

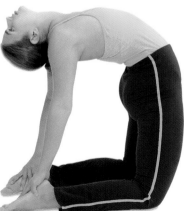

bridge pose
setu bandhasana

Strengthen your body and expand your heart center in this pose.

1 Lie on your back with your knees bent up. Have your knees and feet body-width apart. Lift your pelvis slightly so your buttocks just begin to move off the ground. As you take several breaths in this position, lengthen your tailbone toward your feet. Now peel your vertebrae one by one off the floor. Tuck the shoulders under one by one and move the breastbone toward the chin.

2 A bridge reaches in both directions to the riverbanks. While the breastbone moves toward your chin, the tailbone moves toward the knees and the knees stretch away from you. Don't let your knees splay apart—keep them only as wide as your hips by squeezing the inner thighs toward each other. Check that excess tension is not building up in the neck. After holding five to ten breaths come down and rest. Repeat twice more. Then hug the knees into the chest and rock from side to side to release the back.

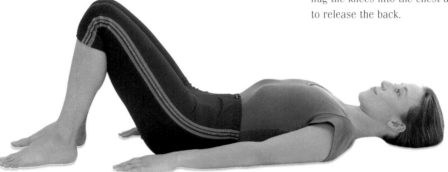

explore*yoga*

If you can straighten your elbows, then interlace the fingers and press the arms down. If your body is ready for more of a challenge, grasp your ankles with your hands. Have patience as you approach each new edge in a pose. Respect the body and wait for it to let you into the pose.

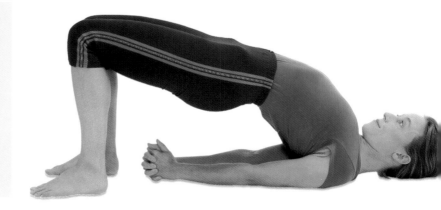

fish pose
matsyasana

This is suitable for releasing the neck after practicing Shoulderstand, Plough, and Knee to Ear pose.

explore*yoga*

Bring your mental sensitivity to the back of the body; feel how it stretches during this pose and the skin thins out.

1 Sit on the floor with your legs in front. For this whole sequence you need to press the insides of the feet and thighs together. Lean back on your hands and pressure the palms to the floor. Lengthen the arms and lift up with the chest. Fully engage your mind in this process. Take your head back and don't forget to breathe. Lift the head and inhale as you come up out of the pose.

2 If you would like to take it a step further, lean back on your elbows so your fingers are by your buttocks. Press down into the elbows and lift the chest into a beautiful arch. With each inhalation, feel the spine move into the core of the body and elongate, setting it up for you to deepen the pose on the exhalation.

3 From position 2, slide your elbows apart to lower down on the crown of your head. Stretch your arms overhead, and reach the fingers away actively. To release, bring the arms to your sides, inhale to lift the head slightly, and then slide it away and lie flat.

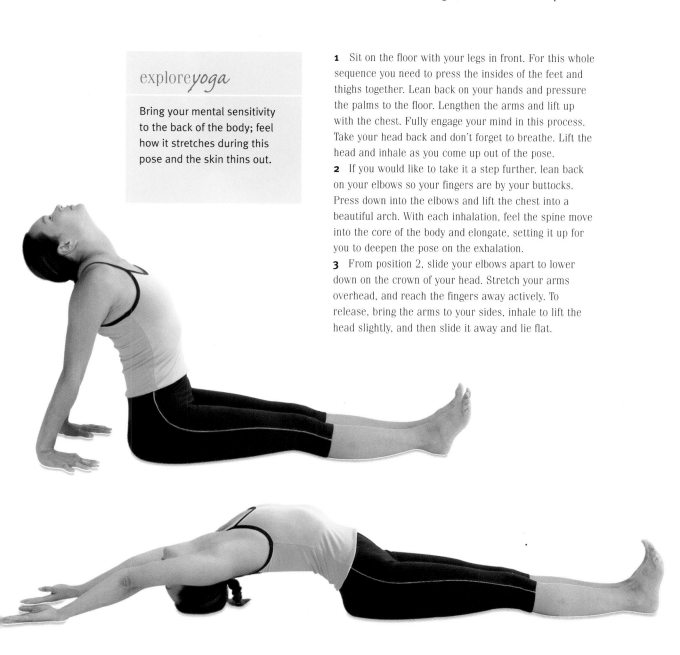

upward-facing bow pose
urdva dhanurasana

Many people who have difficulty rising up into this pose assume that it is because they lack strength, but often it is due to a lack of shoulder flexibility. If your shoulders are tight, then first practice releasing the shoulders with the table prayer pose from the section on alignment (see page 69). Prepare for this with Crescent Moon Pose (see page 70) to open the groin and stretch the thighs.

1   Lie on your back, with your knees bent up. The action on the back is better when the feet are not turned out so check that your toes are pointing forward. Place your palms near the shoulders, fingers pointing in the direction of the hips. Hold here as you allow the anchoring of the heels to earth to take place. Fully feeling the weight of the heels, slowly peel the back up off the floor and lift the hips. Let the grounding of the body come through the heels, then down into the earth.

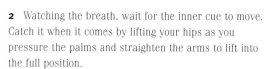

2   Watching the breath, wait for the inner cue to move. Catch it when it comes by lifting your hips as you pressure the palms and straighten the arms to lift into the full position.

3   Now that you are up, adjust your feet, which may have turned out. Press your inner thighs closer together. As in Bridge Pose (see page 74), push the groin up. Let the spine move in toward the front of the body while you consolidate the pose, then expand it in both directions away from the back of the waist. It might help to lengthen toward the tailbone if you lift your heels off the ground for a few breaths.

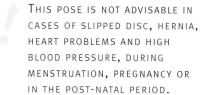

THIS POSE IS NOT ADVISABLE IN CASES OF SLIPPED DISC, HERNIA, HEART PROBLEMS AND HIGH BLOOD PRESSURE, DURING MENSTRUATION, PREGNANCY OR IN THE POST-NATAL PERIOD.

after *backbending*

Always practice a couple of twists and forward bends after a session on backbending.

Sukhasana Twist

As the abdominal muscles contract in this twist, the muscles on the back side of the body can release.

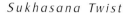

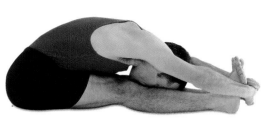

Paschimottanasana

Stretch out the back and hamstrings in this pose.

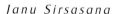

Janu Sirsasana

Janu Sirsasana nicely combines a forward bend with a twisting and lengthening action for each side of the back.

Child Pose— Balasana and Yogamudrasana

These two poses cultivate the sense of release and surrender.

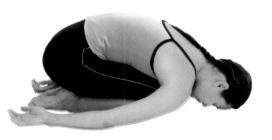

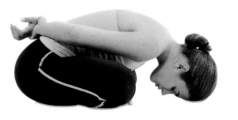

Passive Reclining Twist

Let the softness inherent in this pose release the back.

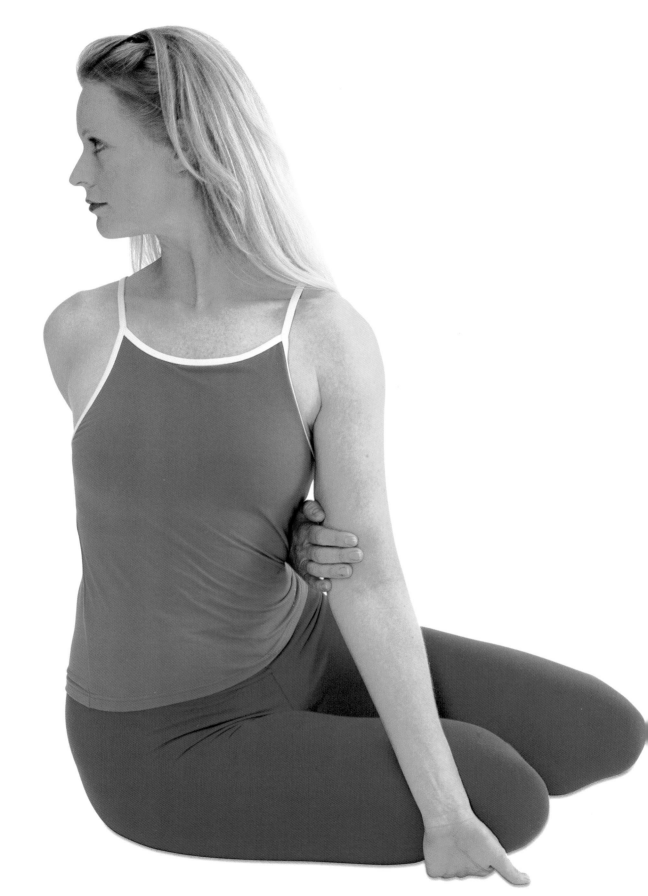

7 Twists

From where you're sitting, twist around to one side for ten breaths. Wind yourself up tight. Coil around with every cell in your torso. Now uncoil. Feel different? A twist is a great opportunity to turn and see things from a different angle.

When you feel wound up by life, temporarily increase the winding with a twist. Spiral up to the sky, then feel the tension dissipate as you undo and consciously unwind out of the twist.

Our well-being depends on a happy spine. Twists prevent stiffness of the spine and counteract any decrease in mobility that makes one look and feel old. Wringing out the body releases lots of built-up tension. Twists can reduce headaches and stiffness in the neck and shoulders. Depending on the cause, they can work miracles in relieving backache, as they stretch and strengthen the tiny muscles that link each vertebra to its neighbour. They help the spine maintain a healthy alignment.

cross-legged twist
pavritta sukhasana

Use this simple cross-legged pose to learn how to twist from bottom to top, and from inside to outside, with awareness.

1 Sit cross-legged and slide your feet crossways so the ankles align under the knees. Bring the heels forward so your shinbones are parallel with each other. Bring the fingertips of the right hand to cup the left knee in front, with those of the left touching the floor behind you.

2 The correct twisting action begins at the root of the back. Learn to work in segments to move the twist progressively up your spine so you can apply the same principles to other twists.

3 Pressure your fingertips down to the floor and inhale yourself taller. To begin the twist, visualize your abdominal organs twisting to the left and, on an exhale, activate the lower abdominal muscles so they move from right to left. On the next exhalation, shunt the middle abdominal muscles left. Visualize an upward spiral of energy. Each time you inhale, feel a further lengthening upward of the spine, and on each exhalation, from the core of the body, twist deeper.

4 When you come to involve the chest in the twist, it works better to twist more on the inhale than the exhale. Remembering to use at least one breath per section, turn the ribs more to the left, then bring the shoulders into the twist. Finally, turn your head left to find the position which feels right for your neck. Hold the pose for five to ten breaths, maintaining the feeling of spinning upward.

5 Unwind and take a moment to feel the effects that the twist has had on your body: sweep over your abdomen, ribs, back, shoulders, and the rest of the body. Check in with your mind too. Twist to the other side, then change the way the legs are crossed and repeat.

Incorrect
Don't jam the floating ribs forward as you bend the spine backward. Keep your back straight so your head and neck are over your pelvis. Both shoulders and both ears should be the same height from the floor.

DON'T PRACTICE TWISTS INTENSIVELY IF YOU HAVE A HERNIA OR HAVE HAD RECENT SURGERY; CONSULT AN EXPERIENCED TEACHER FIRST. PROCEED WITH EXTREME CAUTION IF YOU HAVE DISC PROBLEMS, AS THE TWISTS WILL NEED TO BE IMPLEMENTED GRADUALLY, ALLOWING FOR ANY DELAYED FEEDBACK FROM YOUR BODY. WOMEN BENEFIT FROM PRACTICING TWISTS BETWEEN PERIODS TO RELIEVE MENSTRUAL CRAMPS. DURING MENSTRUATION, USE GENTLE TWISTS. IN PREGNANCY, PRACTICE SIMPLE TWISTS IN AN OPEN WAY (FOR EXAMPLE, WITHOUT COMPRESSING THE ABDOMEN AGAINST THE THIGH) AND FLOW IN AND OUT OF THEM A FEW TIMES WITHOUT HOLDING FOR LONG.

sage twist
bharadvajasana

Spiraling outward and upward releases tension from the whole torso.

1   From Staff Pose (see page 54), bring your legs around to the left and tuck the right foot under the left ankle. Have both knees facing forward. Hold your right knee with your left hand. Bring your right hand to the floor behind you. Sink the sitting bones toward the floor, and take as many breaths as you need to extend up from your base. If this starting position is not comfortable for you, place a small support such as a cushion or folded blanket under one buttock to level yourself off.

2   When you have lengthened well, revolving from the hips, spiral into the fuller twist, moving with the support of your abdominal organs. If possible, slide your left hand under the knee, wrist facing out. Catch hold of your left arm with your right hand and look back over your shoulder. More advanced practitioners can anchor down well through the left sitting bone, allowing the shortened left side of the waist to elongate as the right naturally does. After five to ten breaths, sit on your heels to rest and feel the effects, before repeating on side two.

explore*yoga*

Bring your head into the pose just as you would normally. Measure with your eyes how far around you go. Now turn just your neck and head back to the front. This time, close your eyes, and, with awareness, bring your neck and head back around into the twist. Go only as far as feels healthily comfortable for your neck. Open your eyes and note how far you reached.

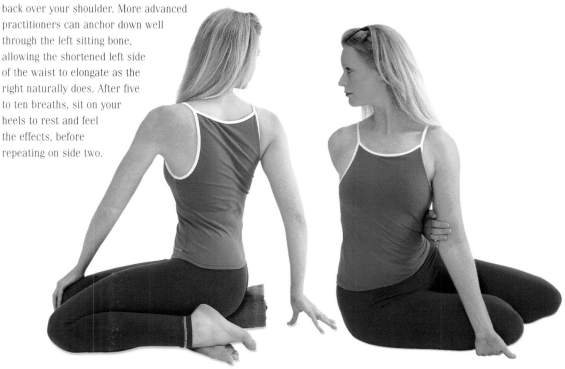

revolved abdomen pose
jathara parivartanasana

Often weak abdominal muscles contribute to chronic back pain. This exercise, practiced daily, will quickly strengthen these muscles. The passive reclining twist in which the floor gives support is less strengthening, but wonderful for easing pain caused by tight back muscles pulling on the vertebrae and causing nerve irritation and pain.

Passive Reclining Twist

1 Lie on your back with your knees bent up close to the chest. Take your arms out to the sides. Keep your knees in close to the body and slowly drop both your knees over to the right side, aiming them toward your elbow. Relax both knees and feet down to the floor. If your knees or feet don't arrive there, rest them on a folded blanket. Turn your head to the left side. There is nothing more to do in this pose. Now bring your attention to actively undoing the parts of the body that are holding on to tension. Check the buttocks, back, shoulders, and face. Stay in this pose for one to two minutes. To come up, turn your head back to center first, lift the top knee in the air, then the other leg, then proceed to side two.

explore*yoga*

You can move the emphasis of the passive twist up and down the back depending on where you place your knees. If your thighs are more at right angles with the torso, the emphasis of the twist is further down the back. If your knees start close to your chest and land close to your elbow, the twist moves up the back.

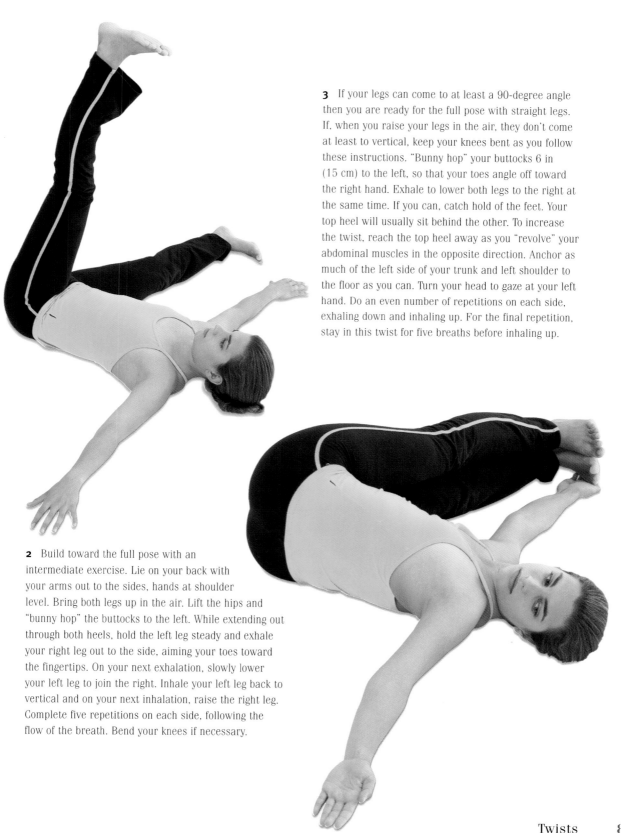

3 If your legs can come to at least a 90-degree angle then you are ready for the full pose with straight legs. If, when you raise your legs in the air, they don't come at least to vertical, keep your knees bent as you follow these instructions. "Bunny hop" your buttocks 6 in (15 cm) to the left, so that your toes angle off toward the right hand. Exhale to lower both legs to the right at the same time. If you can, catch hold of the feet. Your top heel will usually sit behind the other. To increase the twist, reach the top heel away as you "revolve" your abdominal muscles in the opposite direction. Anchor as much of the left side of your trunk and left shoulder to the floor as you can. Turn your head to gaze at your left hand. Do an even number of repetitions on each side, exhaling down and inhaling up. For the final repetition, stay in this twist for five breaths before inhaling up.

2 Build toward the full pose with an intermediate exercise. Lie on your back with your arms out to the sides, hands at shoulder level. Bring both legs up in the air. Lift the hips and "bunny hop" the buttocks to the left. While extending out through both heels, hold the left leg steady and exhale your right leg out to the side, aiming your toes toward the fingertips. On your next exhalation, slowly lower your left leg to join the right. Inhale your left leg back to vertical and on your next inhalation, raise the right leg. Complete five repetitions on each side, following the flow of the breath. Bend your knees if necessary.

passive opening out twist

Stretching out like a starfish expands the heart. Open yourself to a childlike feeling of happiness.

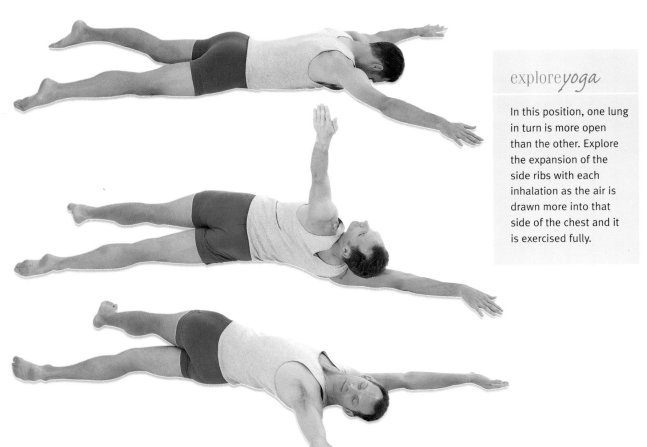

exploreyoga

In this position, one lung in turn is more open than the other. Explore the expansion of the side ribs with each inhalation as the air is drawn more into that side of the chest and it is exercised fully.

1 Lie on your front with your arms and legs apart like a star. Your right hand and both your feet will stay attached to the floor, and your left arm will move.

2 As you bring your arm up and over, let your left hip come up. Allow your knees to bend gently and roll over more onto the sides of your feet. Turn the head to look behind you. Your left arm and shoulder might stay floating in the air. Either use gravity, patience, and the breath to ease them down, or, if you like, rest them on a folded blanket. In time, gravity will assist the easing down process. If your left shoulder can touch the floor, stretch the other shoulder away to increase the distance between them.

3 Rest in this position for one to two minutes, tuning into the purity of the heart center as you do so. Before you move on to do the same on the other side of the body, rest like a starfish to observe what has been mobilized on the physical, mental, and/or emotional levels.

sage pose
marichyasana

This twist develops shoulder flexibility, tones the abdominal organs, and stimulates sluggish intestinal function. This pose is named after the yogi Marichi, who was a man of great wisdom.

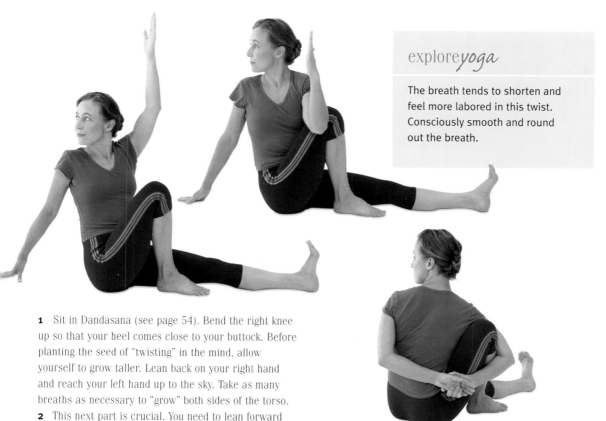

explore *yoga*

The breath tends to shorten and feel more labored in this twist. Consciously smooth and round out the breath.

1 Sit in Dandasana (see page 54). Bend the right knee up so that your heel comes close to your buttock. Before planting the seed of "twisting" in the mind, allow yourself to grow taller. Lean back on your right hand and reach your left hand up to the sky. Take as many breaths as necessary to "grow" both sides of the torso.

2 This next part is crucial. You need to lean forward and wedge your left elbow to the right outer knee without losing the length you have just gained. Do this movement consciously, over one or more exhalations, taking care not to shorten the right side of the torso as you do so. Follow the twisting principals from Cross-Legged Twist (see page 80) to twist in sections from the base up. Feel yourself twisting from the inside out; from the inner organs to the outer casing of your body. Hold the pose for five to ten breaths, then untwist, re-center, and repeat on the other side.

3 For the full posture, straighten your right arm forward. Reach well forward as if you were taking your armpit beyond the right outer knee. From the shoulder, rotate the whole arm so that the thumb turns down, and wrap your arm around the right knee. Clasp the left wrist behind your back, or work your hands toward each other using a soft belt. As you breathe deeply in this pose, the pressure of your thigh against your abdomen gives the organs a healthy massage.

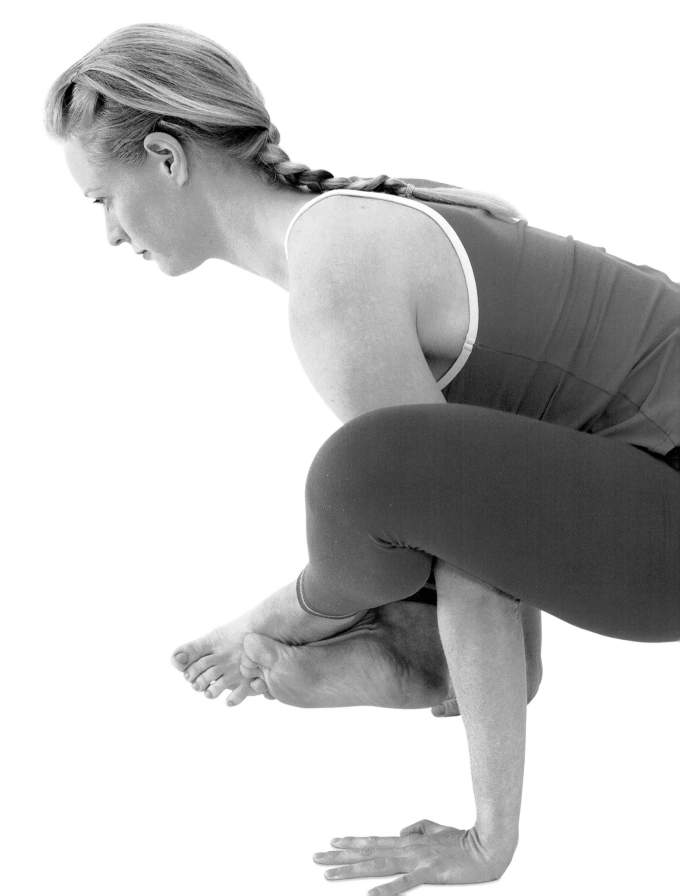

8 Balances

Our lives feel better when they are well balanced. We are healthiest when we find the appropriate balance in our food and we feel best when we find the right levels of activity and sleep. Intellectual balance means we are able to see both sides of the coin, and be less judgmental.

Emotionally, we seek to lessen extremes of emotions, decrease mood swings, and be more even-tempered. Spiritual balance lets us keep higher ideals in mind as our actions create our lives, yet still allows us to keep our feet on the ground. A spiritual belief balances and gives meaning to our physical existence. Being out of balance is a huge source of stress and tends to create problems. Your yoga practice is a metaphor for your life. Finding your balance in a pose is practice at finding your balance in your life. Yoga, as a re-harmonizer, helps you move closer to your own perfect balance.

hand to foot pose
utthita hasta padangusthasana

When a balance pose is a challenge to flexibility,
it is amazing how we are forced to focus to stay up.
This is good practice.

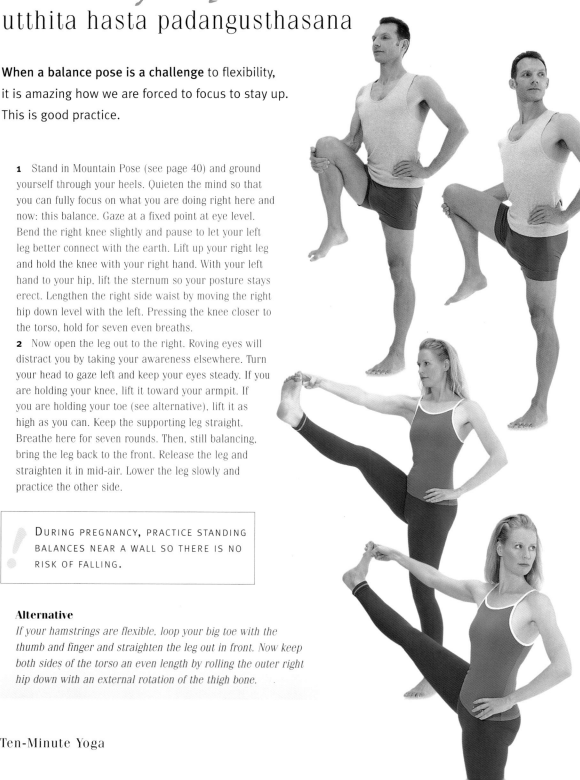

1   Stand in Mountain Pose (see page 40) and ground
yourself through your heels. Quieten the mind so that
you can fully focus on what you are doing right here and
now: this balance. Gaze at a fixed point at eye level.
Bend the right knee slightly and pause to let your left
leg better connect with the earth. Lift up your right leg
and hold the knee with your right hand. With your left
hand to your hip, lift the sternum so your posture stays
erect. Lengthen the right side waist by moving the right
hip down level with the left. Pressing the knee closer to
the torso, hold for seven even breaths.

2   Now open the leg out to the right. Roving eyes will
distract you by taking your awareness elsewhere. Turn
your head to gaze left and keep your eyes steady. If you
are holding your knee, lift it toward your armpit. If
you are holding your toe (see alternative), lift it as
high as you can. Keep the supporting leg straight.
Breathe here for seven rounds. Then, still balancing,
bring the leg back to the front. Release the leg and
straighten it in mid-air. Lower the leg slowly and
practice the other side.

> DURING PREGNANCY, PRACTICE STANDING
> BALANCES NEAR A WALL SO THERE IS NO
> RISK OF FALLING.

Alternative
*If your hamstrings are flexible, loop your big toe with the
thumb and finger and straighten the leg out in front. Now keep
both sides of the torso an even length by rolling the outer right
hip down with an external rotation of the thigh bone.*

eagle pose
garudasana

This pose develops concentration and coordination and is wonderful for tight shoulders.

1 Standing in Mountain Pose (see page 40), become aware of the skin on the soles of the feet as the feet widen out against the floor. Move your attention to the pressure of the right foot against the floor. Quietly let the skin of the foot melt down into it. Then bend the left knee and lift up the right leg.

2 Use momentum to wrap the right leg around the left leg. If you have difficulty with this, bend the supporting leg more. If possible, keep the top knee facing forward, not turned outward. To wrap the arms, hug yourself with your left arm on top of the right. Keeping the cross at the elbows, bring the backs of the hands toward each other, then cross wrist and forearm to bring the palms together.

3 Lift the elbows up so they rise off the chest and free breath is not impeded. To stretch into the shoulders more, ease your forearms forward so your thumbs move away from your nose. Let your eagle fold forward, as if looking down on the world from a great height. When you breathe deeply, you will feel the skin between the shoulder blades stretch on each inhalation. Hold the pose for ten breaths, before unwrapping, re-grounding, and repeating on the opposite side.

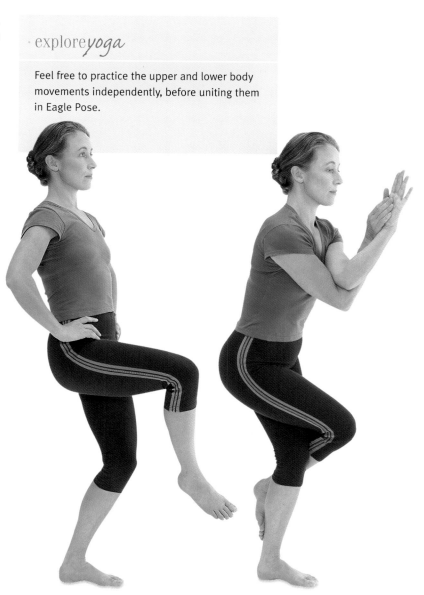

explore*yoga*

Feel free to practice the upper and lower body movements independently, before uniting them in Eagle Pose.

warrior III
virabhadrasana III

Let your warrior-like determination give you a mental surge to charge the body with energy.

1   Assume the pose for Warrior I with your right foot forward (see page 41).

2   Inhale deeply and, on the exhalation, fold your torso over your front leg, lowering your ribs toward your thigh. On a strong inhalation, straighten the right leg and lift the back leg up to parallel with the floor. Gaze straight ahead. Keeping your right leg straight, lower your left hip down so it is even with the right. Turn your left toes from the side down toward the floor and extend back through the heel. (You can even place your hands on the back of a chair to practice the alignment.) Visualize a line of energy running along the body. From the back of the waist it extends forward, reaching out toward the fingertips. From your center, it extends backward through the back heel, so everything from heel to fingertips unkinks and elongates. Hold the pose for five breaths before coming gracefully back to Warrior I.

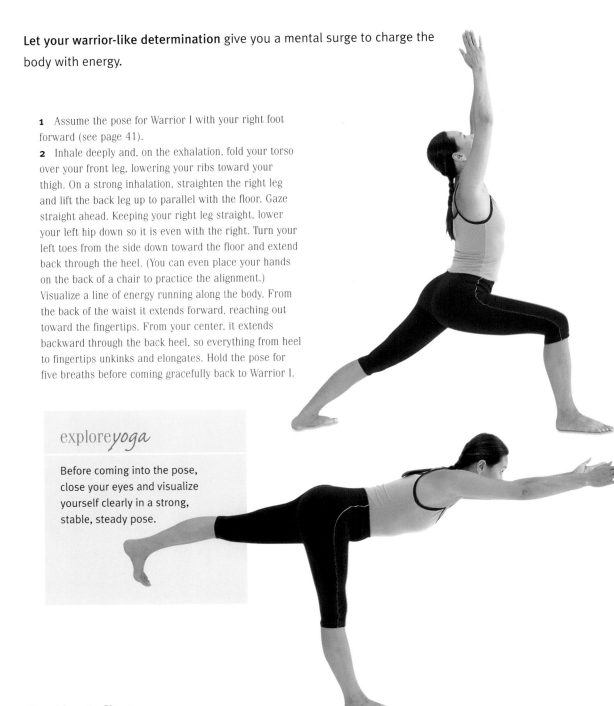

explore*yoga*

Before coming into the pose, close your eyes and visualize yourself clearly in a strong, stable, steady pose.

boat pose
navasana

We can learn the most from the asanas we find the most challenging. By practicing Navasana daily you will notice an increase in abdominal strength within a few weeks.

1 From Staff Pose (see page 54), lean back onto your hands and tilt the pelvis forward. Feel how the vertebral column moves upward and in toward the front of the body. The muscles in the lower back and along the spine engage and the chest lifts. When the stomach muscles work, the belly will naturally bulge a little. However, use this pose to practice an internal energy lock called Uddyana Bandha. Apply this lock by tucking in your lower abdomen, just above the pubic bone and below the navel so it draws closer toward your spine. As you lift your toes in the air, this sucking inward will stop any bulging in the lower abdomen. To go a step further, raise your legs in the air. Practice keeping the inward curve in the lower back, chest lifted and sucking in of the lower abdomen to stop it bulging. Repeat three times, holding for five long breaths.

explore*yoga*

If your back is strong, you can lie on your back with arms overhead and lift up into the final pose in a single movement.

Alternative

To move to a more challenging option, have the knees bent so that the shins are parallel to the floor. Without rounding the back or collapsing the chest, reach the arms toward the toes.

2 In the final pose, keep in mind the principles you practiced initially. Straighten your legs in the air. Adhere the front thigh muscles to the thigh bones, as if they were to tuck up into the torso. This will give you a lift to help prevent any sinking of the chest. Without rounding the back or collapsing the chest, reach your hands forward and gaze up at your big toes.

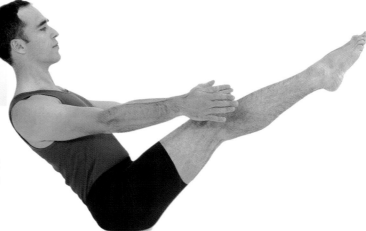

arm pressure balance
bhujapidasana

Despite appearances, this pose doesn't require more upper body strength than you already have. Technique is all-important. With attention to proper positioning and a positive mental attitude you will be well on your way to balancing.

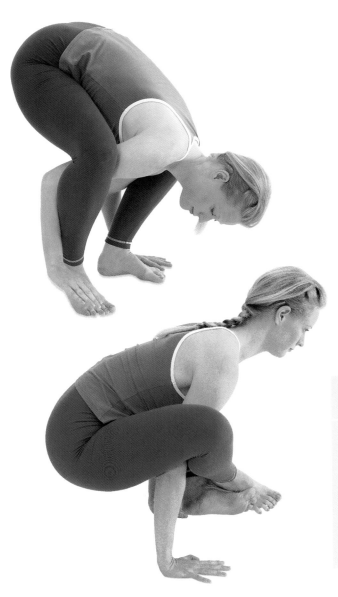

1 Stand with the feet hip-width apart. As you fold forward, bend the knees but keep your hips high in the air. Take the right arm through the legs and around the right leg. A common error is not to take the whole arm—up to the shoulder—through the legs. It is important that the back of the thigh contacts as high up the upper arm as possible so use your other hand to stabilize you if necessary. Place the right palm flat on the floor just next to the right foot with fingers facing forward. Now take the left arm through to bring that palm flat to the floor. You'll need to keep the hips high so you don't squash your upper arm and get stuck halfway in.

2 Bending your elbows well, lean forward. Inch your feet together and forward. Lift up through the abdominal region (see Boat Pose on page 91) and raise your head to gaze forward. Shift your weight to transfer more weight to the palms as you lift your feet up in the air to cross the ankles. Straighten the arms and hold for five to ten breaths. After resting, repeat with the feet crossed the opposite way.

explore*yoga*

Should your wrists need strengthening, practice Downward-Facing Dog (see page 96). To counter-stretch the arms after Arm Pressure Balance, Crane Pose or Downward-Facing Dog, kneel and place the backs of the hands on the floor, fingers facing toward your knees. Move the hips back about 2 in (5 cm). Feel the welcome release along the wrists and forearms as you lean back.

crane pose
bakasana

This pose, resembling a bird, strengthens the upper body and abdomen.

1 Squat with your feet together. Place your hands on the floor as wide as your shoulders, middle fingers facing forward, outer fingers spread. Bend your knees to rest them high up the upper arms, wrapping your inner knees around the upper arms. Bring the feet together and come onto your tiptoes.

2 Lean forward to allow the transfer of weight from toes to palms. Gaze forward along the floor. Lift the abdominal muscles and use yogic energy locks, the bandhas (see page 91), to give your body lift and lightness. One at a time, or together, raise the feet toward the buttocks. Keep your abdominal muscles contracted to help draw the legs into the body. Straighten your arms. Take five breaths before coming down with control.

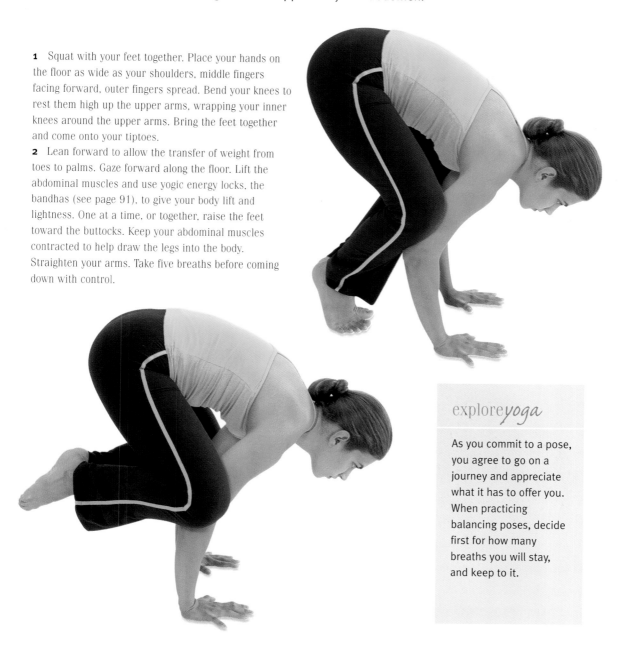

explore*yoga*

As you commit to a pose, you agree to go on a journey and appreciate what it has to offer you. When practicing balancing poses, decide first for how many breaths you will stay, and keep to it.

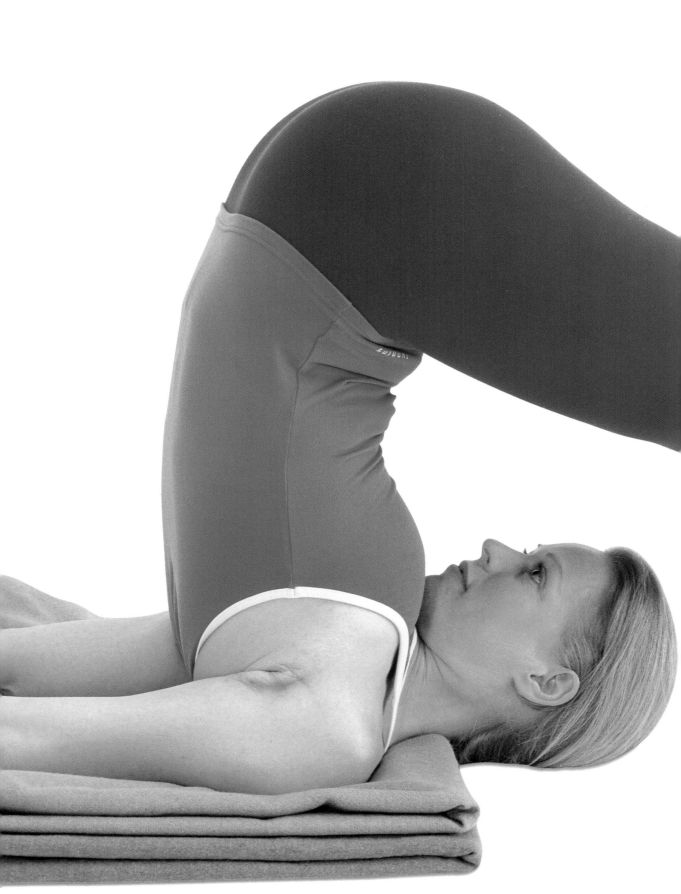

9   Inversions

Holding a position with a whole new relationship to gravity demands a certain steadiness of posture and mind. Inversions develop confidence and help quiet the brain in times of stress.

Inversions are key poses for regaining hormonal balance, as better blood circulation tones the endocrine glands. In particular, Headstand tones the pituitary and pineal glands in the brain, both of which have wide-ranging effects in the body.

When you feel stuck, or in need of inspiration, it helps to see the world from another angle. Releasing the pressure of our normal reality—gravity—can lighten the mind too. Being in an upside-down position gives you a chance to consider things from a different point of view.

Many swear that inversions, through their effects of cleansing and nourishing the tissues, help to maintain youthfulness.

downward-facing dog
adho mukha svanasana

This is an excellent pose for stretching and strengthening the whole body. This forward-folding mild inversion is useful to link standing poses. Although it may not feel very restful at first, it can become so when you develop strength and flexibility. If, instead of being relatively straight, your back rounds in the full Downward-Facing Dog, practice Puppy Dog (opposite). As a gentler way to open the shoulders, you can hold and breathe in this pose longer. If wrist problems prevent you doing the full pose at this time, you should also begin with this easier version.

1 Begin on all fours with your hands placed about 6 in (15 cm) in front of the shoulders. Check that the middle finger is pointing straight ahead, and spread the fingers wide apart.

IF YOU SUFFER HIGH BLOOD PRESSURE, A NECK PROBLEM, EYE, EAR, OR SINUS PROBLEMS, HEART PROBLEMS, HIATUS HERNIA, OR DIZZY SPELLS, SEEK ADVICE FROM A MEDICAL PRACTITIONER OR EXPERIENCED YOGA TEACHER BEFORE BEGINNING INVERSIONS. DURING PREGNANCY, WORK WITH AN EXPERIENCED TEACHER. INVERSIONS ARE NOT NORMALLY ADVISABLE DURING MENSTRUATION, AS THEY TEND TO SLOW THE FLOW OF BLOOD. DON'T PRACTICE INVERTED POSES IF YOU HAVE A HEADACHE AT THE TIME. AS INVERSIONS ARE CONSIDERED TO BE BOTH CALMING TO THE MIND AND COOLING TO THE SYSTEM, THEY ARE GENERALLY USED TOWARD THE END OF LONGER ASANA PRACTICES, AND WHEN YOUR BODY HAS BEEN WARMED BY THE OTHER POSES.

2 Have your knees and feet body width apart. Tuck the toes under and lift up to an inverted "V" position. On tiptoes, bend both knees deeply, so your ribs come toward the thighs, or even touch. You will feel an increase in the stretch through the shoulders and an opening in the chest. At the same time, lift the sitting bones as the buttocks stay high and tilt the pelvis forward. The inward curve in the lower back will deepen as your navel moves closer to your thighs. (This pose is also a forward bend, so refresh your body's memory about folding from the hips: see page 46.) You will feel the muscles along the spine working strongly and get a lifting sense of elongation along the spine.

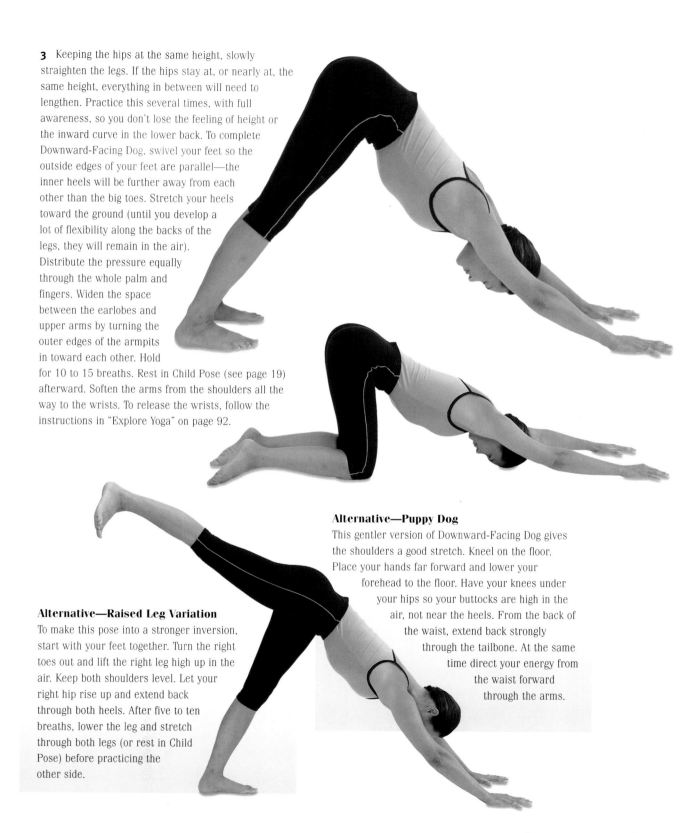

3 Keeping the hips at the same height, slowly straighten the legs. If the hips stay at, or nearly at, the same height, everything in between will need to lengthen. Practice this several times, with full awareness, so you don't lose the feeling of height or the inward curve in the lower back. To complete Downward-Facing Dog, swivel your feet so the outside edges of your feet are parallel—the inner heels will be further away from each other than the big toes. Stretch your heels toward the ground (until you develop a lot of flexibility along the backs of the legs, they will remain in the air). Distribute the pressure equally through the whole palm and fingers. Widen the space between the earlobes and upper arms by turning the outer edges of the armpits in toward each other. Hold for 10 to 15 breaths. Rest in Child Pose (see page 19) afterward. Soften the arms from the shoulders all the way to the wrists. To release the wrists, follow the instructions in "Explore Yoga" on page 92.

Alternative—Puppy Dog

This gentler version of Downward-Facing Dog gives the shoulders a good stretch. Kneel on the floor. Place your hands far forward and lower your forehead to the floor. Have your knees under your hips so your buttocks are high in the air, not near the heels. From the back of the waist, extend back strongly through the tailbone. At the same time direct your energy from the waist forward through the arms.

Alternative—Raised Leg Variation

To make this pose into a stronger inversion, start with your feet together. Turn the right toes out and lift the right leg high up in the air. Keep both shoulders level. Let your right hip rise up and extend back through both heels. After five to ten breaths, lower the leg and stretch through both legs (or rest in Child Pose) before practicing the other side.

headstand/hare pose
sirsasana/sasankasana

Your head weighs about 9 lb (4 kg), your body considerably more. Your neck can hold the weight of your body only when you are properly prepared. It is essential to understand the lifting through the shoulders and pay due attention to alignment. This is not a beginners' pose and I strongly recommend you ask an experienced teacher to observe your alignment. If Headstand is not yet for you, the Hare Pose is a possible alternative.

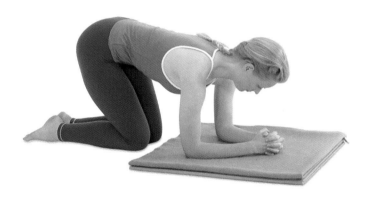

1 Always practice Headstand on a cushioned surface such as a folded blanket. Place your blanket in front of a wall, or in the corner of two walls. Kneel in front of your blanket. To measure out the correct elbow width, place your forearms on the blanket, and cup each elbow in the opposite hand. Your elbows should be not wider than your shoulders. Then form your triangle of support by interlacing your fingers together. Your knuckles should be 2 in (5 cm) from the wall.

2 When performing a safe Headstand, it is crucial to lift well from elbows to shoulders. Tuck your toes under and straighten your knees so you are in an inverted "V" shape. Practice your lift by pressing down through the elbows and moving the shoulders up toward the hips. This movement should increase the distance between the shoulders and earlobes as well as lifting the head away from the floor. If you find you can't lift your head away from the floor, you are not ready for Headstand yet. You need to develop your shoulder flexibility and/or strength before attempting to go up into Headstand. For shoulder flexibility, practice the shoulder exercises on page 69, as well as Gomukhasana (see page 64), and Garudasana (see page 89). To develop arm strength, practice Downward-Facing Dog (see page 96).

3 Take your knees back to the floor and position your head on the floor to be cupped by your interlaced fingers. For the correct alignment in the neck, it is the crown of the head that should be in contact with the floor. Once again raise the knees off the floor and practice moderating the pressure on the head.

Ground down through the elbows, distribute weight into the edges of the hands against the floor, lift the shoulders up toward the hips. If you are not able to minimize the pressure on the crown of the head with these actions, then don't move onto the next step. Develop this skill with some more preparatory work before you come up into Headstand.

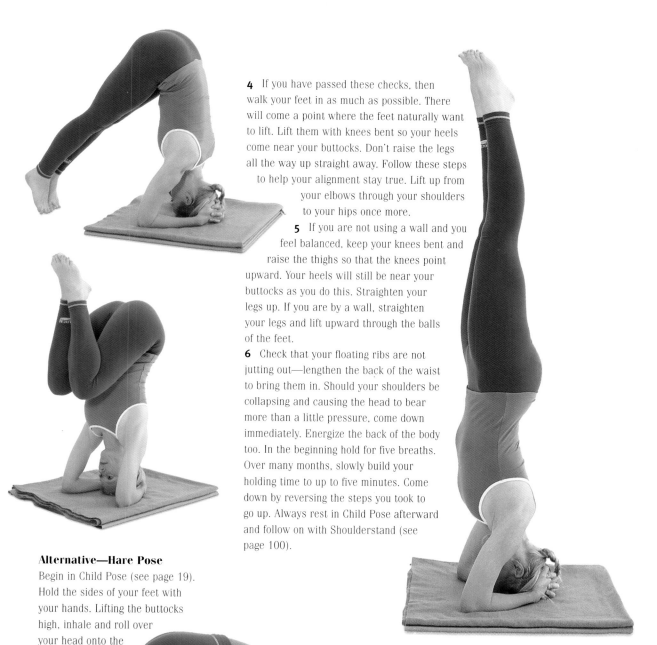

4 If you have passed these checks, then walk your feet in as much as possible. There will come a point where the feet naturally want to lift. Lift them with knees bent so your heels come near your buttocks. Don't raise the legs all the way up straight away. Follow these steps to help your alignment stay true. Lift up from your elbows through your shoulders to your hips once more.

5 If you are not using a wall and you feel balanced, keep your knees bent and raise the thighs so that the knees point upward. Your heels will still be near your buttocks as you do this. Straighten your legs up. If you are by a wall, straighten your legs and lift upward through the balls of the feet.

6 Check that your floating ribs are not jutting out—lengthen the back of the waist to bring them in. Should your shoulders be collapsing and causing the head to bear more than a little pressure, come down immediately. Energize the back of the body too. In the beginning hold for five breaths. Over many months, slowly build your holding time to up to five minutes. Come down by reversing the steps you took to go up. Always rest in Child Pose afterward and follow on with Shoulderstand (see page 100).

Alternative—Hare Pose

Begin in Child Pose (see page 19). Hold the sides of your feet with your hands. Lifting the buttocks high, inhale and roll over your head onto the crown. On the exhalation, release back to Child Pose. Repeat five times.

> **!** HEADSTAND, SHOULDERSTAND, HALASANA, AND KARNAPIDASANA SHOULD NOT BE PRACTICED DURING MENSTRUATION OR WITH CERTAIN EAR OR EYE PROBLEMS, SUCH AS DETACHED RETINA OR GLAUCOMA. FOR HEART PROBLEMS, HIGH BLOOD PRESSURE, PREVIOUS NECK INJURIES, OR PREGNANCY, SEEK THE ADVICE OF AN EXPERIENCED TEACHER.

shoulderstand
sarvangasana

This hormone-balancing and deeply calming pose is well worth practicing daily.

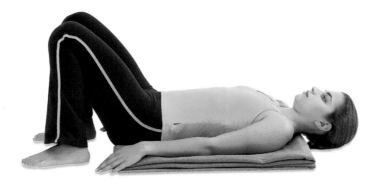

1 To enable you to keep your neck relaxed in this pose, fold two or three blankets to the size that will support your base. Place the folded edges neatly one on top of the other. Lie over them with your head on the lower level, and the tops of your shoulders on your blankets, 2 in (5 cm) from the edge.

2 With control, bring your legs and hips in the air and then support your back. If your stomach muscles are not yet strong enough to bring you up, or if you can't yet come up in a well-controlled way that feels safe, use the wall method (see opposite). Once you are up, bend your knees toward your head. Take several breaths to settle your shoulders into the pose. Let yourself come more onto the tips of the well-grounded shoulders and walk the hands down your back. Finally, stretch your legs up into the air. In the beginning, your legs may be angled to be quite bent overhead, not straight up in the air. Bring your elbows closer together. You may get a better grip holding your palms against the skin on your back rather than your clothes. In time, work on lessening the crease where the thighs join the torso. Visualize a line of energy from the inner thigh to the inner heel.

3 Never turn the head from side to side in this pose. Shoulderstand is not called neckstand for good reason! Although it might look like the neck is taking a lot of weight, the neck muscles need to stay relatively soft. If possible, ask a friend to touch the muscles on either side of your neck to check they are not strained tight. Likewise, redness or strain in the face means it's time to come down and rest. Build your time in the pose from one to up to 10 minutes.

4 After Shoulderstand, you can practice Halasana or Karnapidasana (pages 102 and 103). To come down, use the abdominal muscles to lower yourself down in a slow, controlled way. Slide off the blankets and lie flat. Release your neck by turning your head from side to side. The lower back and abdominal organs will probably communicate some different sensations to you, so practice with a twist and a forward bend afterward.

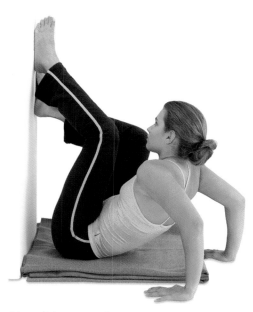

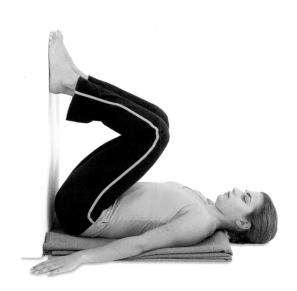

Shoulderstand Against the Wall

This controlled, step-by-step way of lifting into
Shoulderstand in stages is a good way to start feeling
comfortable with Shoulderstand.

1 Place your folded blankets a little away from the
wall—as your head needs to be off the blankets but
your shoulders supported by them, you may have to
experiment to find the correct width for the length of
your body. If you have a non-slip yoga mat, place it on
top of the blankets. Sit side on and up close to the wall.
Using your arms for support, slowly bring your legs up
the wall and move your trunk around and down until you
are lying over the blankets.

2 If you have found the right position with your blankets,
your head will be on the floor, your shoulders 2 in
(5 cm) from the edge of the blankets, and your buttocks
near the wall. Lift your head and check that your body
is symmetrical, perpendicular to the wall.

3 Now you are ready to come up! With knees bent, press
your feet into the wall and lift your hips. Hold your back
and straighten yourself up by moving your hips more in
line over your shoulders. If you like, you can straighten
each leg in turn bringing one foot up the wall. Once you
have both legs straight against the wall, take one leg,
then the other, overhead and away from the wall. Come
down by reversing the steps you took to go up.

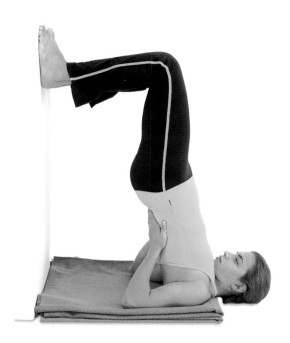

> **!** FOR CONTRAINDICATIONS TO
> SHOULDERSTAND, SEE PAGE 99.

plough pose
halasana

If you are comfortable in Shoulderstand, follow on with this soothing pose. It has similar effects and contraindications to Shoulderstand.

1 From Shoulderstand lower your legs overhead. You need to be careful not to overstretch the neck as you bring your toes to touch the floor. If you are not able to bring your toes to the floor, then rest them on a higher surface, such as a chair placed a couple of feet behind the head. (If your toes are not supported, then continue to support your back with your hands.)

2 Once your toes are resting on a surface, stretch your arms along the floor. This will help you roll more onto the tips of your shoulders and deeper into this upside-down forward bend. Interlace your fingers and deepen the pose by stretching your arms and legs in opposite directions. Gradually build up until you can hold this pose for five minutes. Make Plough Pose more restful by supporting the thighs with a chair.

3 Roll out of the pose with control, using your abdominal muscles to lower both legs until you are lying flat. See Shoulderstand for complementary asanas to follow on with.

> ! FOR CONTRAINDICATIONS TO HALASANA SEE PAGE 99.

Rollings—From Halasana to Paschimottanasana

You can enjoy a lovely massage for the muscles along the spine by rolling between Halasana and Paschimottanasana. If you are very comfortable in Plough Pose, lie on a cushioned surface, and use a little momentum and a lot of abdominal strength to roll slowly between these two positions. Inhale as you roll up and back to Halasana and exhale as you roll forward to Paschimottanasana.

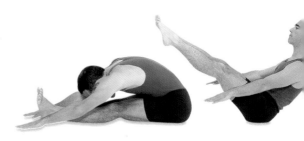

knee to ear pose
karnapidasana

Withdraw into a fetal position after practicing Shoulderstand and Plough Pose.

If you feel comfortable in Halasana, practice this deep forward stretch by cushioning yourself with a couple of folded blankets and bending your knees beside your head. If your knees and tops of the feet don't come to the floor, place your legs on raised supports or tuck your toes under if necessary. To deepen the pose, straighten both arms along the floor and interlace your fingers. If your knees touch the floor, fold your arms over the backs of your knees. Hold this pose for 10 to 20 breaths before coming back to Halasana.

> ❗ FOR CONTRAINDICATIONS TO KARNAPIDASANA, SEE PAGE 99.

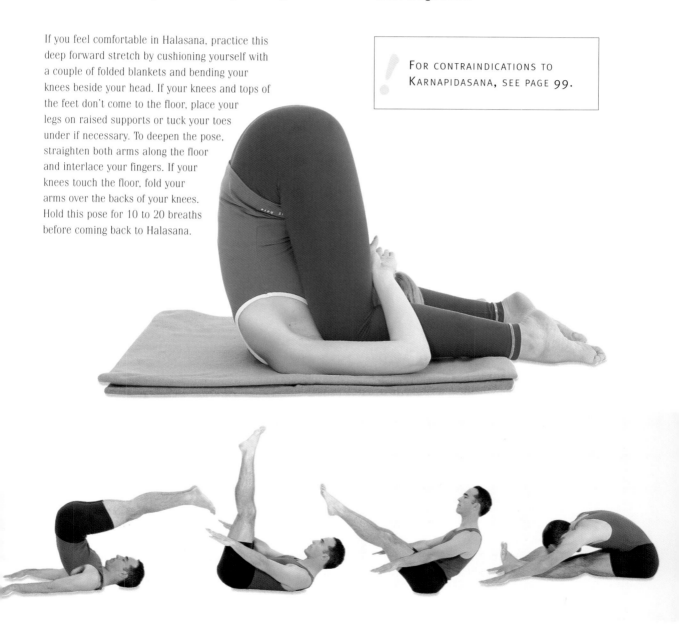

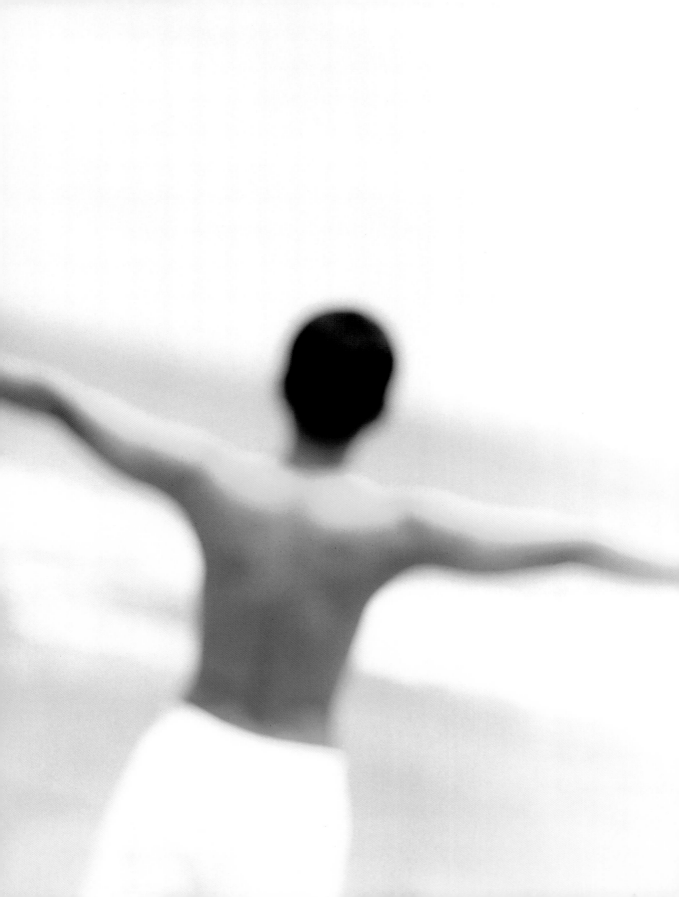

10 YogaBreathing

Have you ever watched children in the playground and marvelled at their never-ending energy? Have you ever felt that you were more tired than you should have been—as if the equation of energy expenditure versus remaining energy didn't add up?

People usually nominate food as the provider of our energy but we forget about a couple of other important sources. Ideas, for one, supply us with boundless energy. You may have experienced being so taken with an idea that you were able to work late into the night without feeling fatigued. A third energy source, recognized by yogis for millennia, is the breath.

Breath, life, and energy are rooted together and yogis have a single word for all three—prana. When pranic levels are high, the body will be completely charged with energy. Pranayama may be translated either as restraint or control of the breath, or as pranic capacity. Pranayama exercises use breathing techniques to increase vitality and mental focus, and also as a means of expanding consciousness.

about *breathing*

Increase the depth of your next inhalation by about 30 percent and observe what happens to your shoulders. If you find that your shoulders lift more than a little, you are probably breathing less efficiently than you could.

The shoulders lift due to the actions of the muscles around the neck and collarbone. In helping us breathe, they should act as accessory muscles only. Overusing them is not an efficient way to get energy from air, so shoulder movement should account for a relatively small percentage of the effort used to inhale.

The most important muscles in your body for breathing are those of the abdominal wall, the little muscles between the ribs, and the diaphragm. The diaphragm, being an internal muscle and harder to access, is less well understood. Something like a trampoline, it spans the width of the mid-torso, separating the chest and abdominal cavities. When this large muscle is relaxed, it curves upward like an upside-down soup bowl. Every time you inhale, it contracts, and the concavity changes as this dome-shaped muscle moves downward. This downward movement increases the space in the chest cavity, which creates a vacuum so that the spongy tissue of the lungs can draw in air from outside.

When you exhale, the diaphragm releases its contraction and moves up, reducing the size of the chest cavity and letting the air flow out of the lungs. The downward movement of the diaphragm (inhalation) increases pressure on the organs in the abdominal cavity. The upward movement (exhalation) releases the pressure. This increase and release of pressure directly affects the health of the abdominal organs. As the diaphragm moves between its downward contraction and upward relaxation, the organs are gently moved and massaged. The rhythm of the breath and free movement of the diaphragm encourage the natural pulsation that healthy organs require.

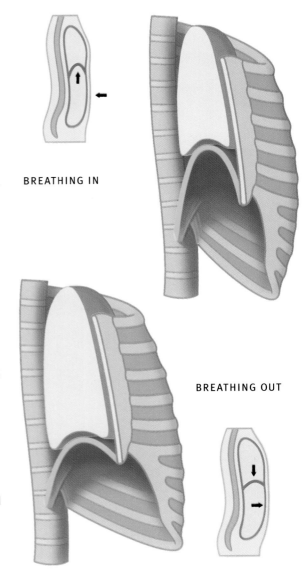

BREATHING IN

BREATHING OUT

how to *sit*

Our bodies are as individual as our personalities, so no single position reigns supreme for pranayama or meditation. There are really only two rules for sitting. The first is to sit erect so that your head, neck, and back are in line. The second is to be perfectly comfortable. Any physical discomfort will interfere with your concentration, alter your breath, and undo a little of your good work.

Comfortable Pose— Sukhasana

Before practicing the cross-legged postures, use the leg cradling warm up (see page 58) to unwind the leg at the hip socket. For Sukhasana, sit cross-legged and slide your feet apart so that each foot comes to rest underneath the opposite knee. It is difficult to sit upright with your shoulders over your hips if your knees are much higher than your hips. Use cushions or folded blankets to raise your seat if necessary.

Perfect Pose—Siddhasana

Sit on a cushioned surface. Fold one leg in so the heel touches to the perineum—the area between the anus and the genitals. Bend the second leg and bring the heel of that foot level with the first one. Rest the backs of your hands on your knees.

Firm Pose—Vajarsana

Kneel with your knees and ankles together and sit down on your heels. As you bring your weight down, your inner ankles will tend to splay apart. Keep them as close together as possible. If it causes discomfort for the tops of the feet, place a small rolled blanket under them. If you like, you can place a folded blanket over your heels before sitting down.

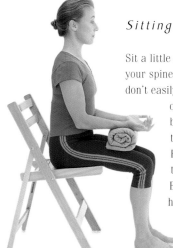

Sitting in a Chair

Sit a little away from the backrest so your spine will be straight. If your feet don't easily touch the ground, rest them on a rolled blanket or telephone book. Fold a blanket several times to make a long pad. Experiment with it lying across the knees in any of these poses. By placing the backs of your hands on the support, your elbows will bend more and softness will come into the palms.

discovering the *breath*

Become aware of your breath. Maintain this awareness until you have finished reading this introduction.

We don't have to think to breathe; it is instinctive and happens automatically. The breath is usually under the control of the medulla oblongata in the relatively primitive brain stem. During pranayama breathing it shifts from being an involuntary and automatic process toward being more of a voluntary one, and it seems this activates the cerebral cortex, a more evolved part of the brain. Pranayama, by bringing a voluntary element to this involuntary process, has profound physiological, psychological and spiritual effects.

Most simply, a breath is an intake of oxygen that gets distributed to our cells. The efficient, natural breath ensures that every cell in your body receives the energy it needs to do its job: digest, grow, heal, detoxify. Logically, a healthy body will be composed of well-nourished cells. Deep, conscious breathing which fully expands the lungs has an enormously positive impact on health and enhances all cellular processes. When we breathe better, we feel better.

When you touch a baby's belly, or a kitten's or puppy's, you can feel the whole torso moving completely freely. The chest and belly open and blossom with each breath. There is a delightful inner pulsation from expansion to consolidation, a sense of real freedom. However, as we move through the process of life, we inevitably sustain some blows. Particularly as children, we have a limited capacity to understand. In response to the impacts of life, we form shielding patterns in our bodies. At some points, in some areas, our breath ceases to be the joyfully free flow it once was, and deviates into a new protective pattern. As adults we still breathe automatically and unconsciously, but due to our reactions to life, few of us breathe optimally. Those energetic children we were watching in the playground most likely still have relatively free breathing, responsive to the natural cues of the body.

Everything we do is affected by our breathing. The breath and the mind are intrinsically related; they are two expressions of the same entity. Think of the last time you felt angry or fearful: your breath became fast, shallow, and irregular. Compare this to when you were dozing in a comfortable chair. Probably your breath was deeper and slower. Just as your mind affects the breath, your breath affects the mind. Yogis have long recognized that when the breath becomes calm, the mind will too. The *Hatha Yoga Pradipika*, an ancient text, tells us, "Respiration being disturbed, the mind becomes disturbed. By restraining respiration (pranayama) the Yogi attains steadiness of the mind."

The breath is a bridge to our nervous system, and

enhanced breathing can improve our mental and emotional states. Firstly, by simply observing our breathing we gain a mental point of focus that can quiet the constant chatter of the mind. Secondly, it relaxes the mind to promote clear, steady thinking, decrease emotional fluctuations, and provide a sense of well-being. It is a valuable tool for self-management. Thirdly, like meditation, pranayama draws the senses inward, deepens awareness, and expands consciousness.

Conscious breathing encourages conscious action and conscious living in a calmer way. For returning to the self, we have been given the miracle of the breath. A good breathing habit is a wonderful ally in life, a valuable tool for self-management when dealing with confrontations, fear, agitation, anger and confusion.

Conscious breathing is certainly a mental challenge. Did you remember to be aware of your breath just now, even as you were sitting reading?

Voluntary control of the breath helps to cast off accumulated stress as well as improving lung capacity.

explore*yoga*

The exercises fall into two categories. During exercises in returning to the natural breath (see pages 28 and 110) you immerse yourself in your true breath and begin to disentangle it from any other superimposed breathing patterns. These exercises, where you don't add anything to your breath, are a great starting place. Release any pressure you may feel to breathe "correctly" or do it "the right way" and let your instincts take over. You can repeat them every day for weeks or months to get to know your breath, and return to them as often as you wish. The remaining exercises are pranayama, some of which lead on to more advanced practices involving alteration of the breath. If you wish to develop these practices further, the best way is to work alongside an experienced teacher.

Breath awareness and pranayama are fundamental and they should be practised daily. Just a few minutes will still be worthwhile. Use Savasana relaxation (see page 20) to separate pranayama and asana practice so that your energies settle.

VERY DEEP INHALATIONS SHOULD NOT BE PRACTICED IF YOU HAVE HYPERTENSION OR HEART PROBLEMS. EXTREMELY LONG EXHALATIONS ARE NOT ADVISABLE IF YOU SUFFER FROM LOW BLOOD PRESSURE OR DEPRESSION.

breathing in all *directions*

This exercise is usually done with a partner, but can also be done alone. In position 1, lightly place your own hands where the partner's hands would be. In position 2, let your shoulders slide up and elbows fall down towards the floor as you curl your palms around your sides. In position 3, let your elbows and shoulders be as heavy and relaxed as possible as you place your hands on your back ribs. Helpers can direct their breath to the same areas as their partner.

Breathing into the Front

1 Lie on your back with your knees bent and feet flat on the floor. With feet wider than hips, lean your knees together. Helpers need to be sitting perfectly comfortably so they can hold the position for the duration. Any tension will spill over to their partner. Your helper places one palm over your navel and the other high up on the chest, from just below the notch at the base of the throat, using a light touch to increase awareness. When you are comfortable, have your partner read the instructions to you with generous pauses after each sentence to allow you to explore.

2 Close your eyes. Observe how your body moves with each inhalation. Which part of your body moves first? Can you feel where the breath originates? What happens next? Observe the sequence of movement. What happens to the lower and upper abdomen? How does the rib cage alter? And the chest? Which part feels like it expands more? Let the breath move you. What happens to the shoulders, the throat? Is there any tightness or constriction there? What about the face and nostrils?

3 Now turn your attention to the out breath. From where does your exhalation begin? Where does your exhalation end? Are the movements in the torso as clearly demarcated as in your inhalation? There is a yielding quality to the exhalation, a slow release as the body softens down into the floor. Can you feel a sort of consolidation in toward the center of your torso as you exhale? Could it be that the exhalation ends prematurely? Can you extend the exhalation by being patient and not rushing on to the next breath?

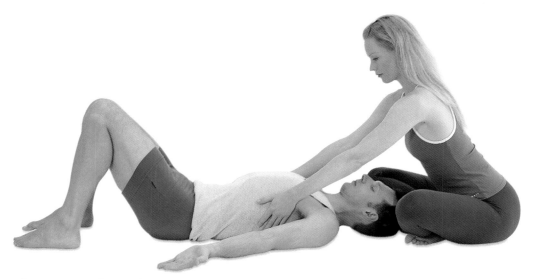

Breathing into the Sides

1 Maintain the quiet stillness as your partner changes position to hold the side ribs, cupping just under the armpits. Observe the horizontal expansion of the ribs on the inhalation; the outward and upward movement each time you draw air in. If you don't feel much movement, exhale more fully so that the inhalation naturally deepens. Observe how each exhalation brings a downward and inward movement.

2 Now pay attention to the timing of these movements in relation to your abdomen and chest. As you inhale, you might find the abdomen expands first, then the side ribs move up and out, and finally the upper chest expands. If this movement is difficult to isolate, then you should momentarily try to deepen your breathing so that you can discover your particular breathing pattern. What is your pattern of breathing out? Can you isolate the order of the movement of the abdomen, side ribs and chest or do they all seem to run together?

Breathing into the Back

1 Keeping your mental focus, kneel and fold forward into Child Pose. You need to be completely comfortable, so for modifications of the posture, see page 19. Your partner places their hands just below your shoulder blades, fingers wrapping around the sides.

2 Take your breath to the back of your body. Mentally direct the air into your partner's hands. As if you had little balloons under your partner's hands, feel your inhalation "puff" out against them. Have patience as you wait for the movement to come. Many people find this rather difficult and you may find that developing this awareness may take several practices.

3 In the beginning, you might find it helpful to limit your breathing into the front of the torso by slightly holding in the part of the abdomen below the navel. Visualize the breath moving into the back of the body. As well, have your partner press in slightly during your exhalation to remind you where to expand out to on the inhalation. Once you begin to get a feeling for it, feel the whole back come alive. It opens and blossoms with each inhalation, before softening down on each exhalation.

humming bee breath
bhramari

Making sounds is a great way to bring constancy to the breath. It also lengthens the exhalation, which will naturally deepen the inhalation and encourage a slow, rhythmic breath. Don't be shy of making a sound out loud. The sound provides a point of focus for the mind. As the *Hatha Yoga Pradipika* states, "By this practice one becomes lord of the yogis and the mind is absorbed in bliss." Lose yourself in the vibrations and simply enjoy the soothing effect of Bhramari on the mind.

1 Sit comfortably erect or lie with your knees bent up. Have your mouth closed, jaw relaxed and the teeth slightly apart. Pressing your tongue lightly to the roof of the mouth will create a slight tension and turn the simple humming more into a bee-like droning.

2 Inhale fully, then exhale while making a humming sound. The vocal cords keep just a small amount of tension so the pitch is low. The constancy of the exhalation keeps the sound uniform. The vibration comes from the soft palate at the top of the back of the mouth. Widen the inside of the mouth to increase the resonance in the nasal cavity. Hone your awareness of the vibration to expand it out to the throat, to the top of the head, and eventually the rest of the body. Practice Bhramari for two minutes and build to five. Afterward, sit or lie quietly with eyes closed to enjoy the after-effects. Should you experience dizziness or tingling or should your mind become agitated, switch to simple breathing.

3 Another position for practice is sitting on a blanket with your knees bent up in front of you. Place your elbows on your knees so you can easily cover your eyes with your hands and the flap over your ear holes with your thumbs. Become absorbed in the sound that seems to fill the skull.

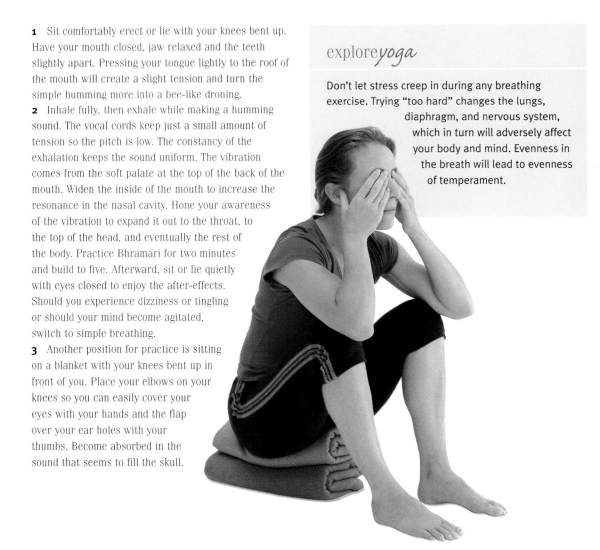

explore*yoga*

Don't let stress creep in during any breathing exercise. Trying "too hard" changes the lungs, diaphragm, and nervous system, which in turn will adversely affect your body and mind. Evenness in the breath will lead to evenness of temperament.

victorious breath

ujjayi pranayama

Uj comes from the word for "up" and jaya means "triumph" or "conquest." Become victorious over any imbalance in the upward-moving prana with Ujjayi breathing. As you grow comfortable with Ujjayi breathing, use if for the duration of your asana practice.

Ujjayi breathing is a little like drinking air through a straw. The glottis lies just behind the larynx, near the male Adam's apple. It's the part of the throat that closes when you gargle or hold your breath. As the air flows past the partially closed glottis, friction is produced. This friction increases heat in the body, allowing it to stretch more than it otherwise would during yoga asana practice. Ujjayi breathing thins the breath, giving control over the flow of air into the lungs so that the breath becomes steadier, deeper, and longer. More oxygen is made available, enhancing the purification and nourishment of each and every cell.

1 Sit in your meditative position. Breathe in through the nose and out through the mouth. Each time you exhale, make a long "haaaa" sound through your mouth, as if you were trying to fog up a mirror.
2 After several cycles, close your mouth midway through an exhalation, but continue to make the "haaaa" with your lips together. It will become a soft sound like a "hm" that you can feel vibrating in the back of the throat. To check if you've got it, cover your ears with your palms and listen to the internal throaty exhalation sound. It will sound like the swish of the ocean.
3 Now bring the sound into the inhalation. Open your mouth again and make this "haaaa" sound as you draw in the air through your mouth. Close your mouth midway through to experience the soft, throaty friction again. When you feel you have got it, cover your ears to check the ocean-like quality of the sound.
4 Now you are ready for the continuous internal 'hm' breathing with your mouth closed. At first, practice Ujjayi for 10 to 20 breaths while sitting. Take breaks to return to your natural breath whenever you need. This

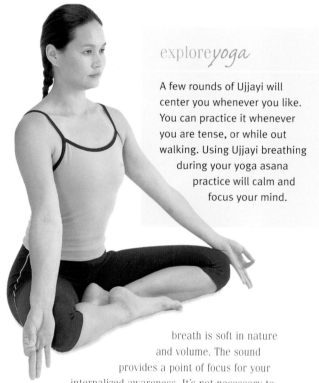

explore yoga

A few rounds of Ujjayi will center you whenever you like. You can practice it whenever you are tense, or while out walking. Using Ujjayi breathing during your yoga asana practice will calm and focus your mind.

breath is soft in nature and volume. The sound provides a point of focus for your internalized awareness. It's not necessary to breathe loudly or aggressively. While the sound produced is audible to someone close by, it's not necessary to fill the whole room. Measure the quality of your Ujjayi breathing, not by volume, but by length and steadiness. Bring your awareness to the constancy that this breath gives you. There should be no surges in the breath, in or out. It should be clean, even and pleasant. Each inhalation extends in a long, fluid way to completely fill the lungs. Likewise, the flow of air outward through your nostrils is slow and steady for the entire duration of the exhalation.

alternate nostril breathing
nadi suddhi pranayama

This exercise acts as a purification (suddhi) of the subtle energy meridians (the nadis). As it helps balance the nervous system, it is useful when you feel uptight or confused. It calms the mind yet leaves you mentally alert. Practice after a hard day at work, when you feel fearful, or before bed to quiet the mind for sleep.

1 Sit comfortably. Curl the index and middle fingers of your right hand into the palm. Inhale fully through both nostrils.

2 Close the right nostril with the thumb of the right hand and exhale fully through the left nostril.

3 Still keeping the right thumb covering the right nostril, now inhale through the left side.

4 Close the left nostril with your ring and little finger.

5 Release your thumb and exhale through the right nostril.

6 Inhale through the right side.

7 Close the right nostril and exhale through the left.

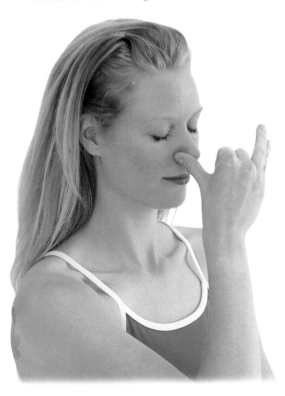
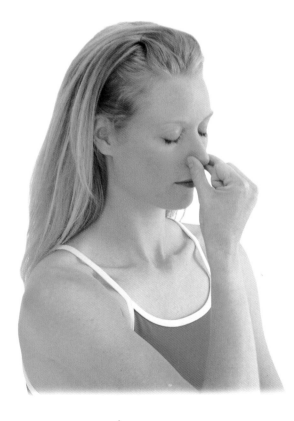

This is one cycle. Complete three to seven cycles before resting your arm down, and breathing quietly through both nostrils. Wait until you feel ready before starting the next round. Complete three to seven rounds and finish by relaxing in Savasana (see page 20).

The air moves through the nostrils at a constant rate. From beginning to end, during each inhalation and exhalation, the air flows at the same speed. There is no strain and the breath will have a soft quality. Visualize a saucer of fine wood ash just under your nose. If you inhale too greedily the ash would be sucked inside your nose. If you exhale forcefully, it would end up settling over your clothes.

During the practice, keep your right elbow raised to avoid placing pressure on your chest and impeding the lungs from filling. Tension can build up in the shoulder and arm so change hands as necessary. Open your eyes occasionally to check that your head is straight, not tilted off to one side.

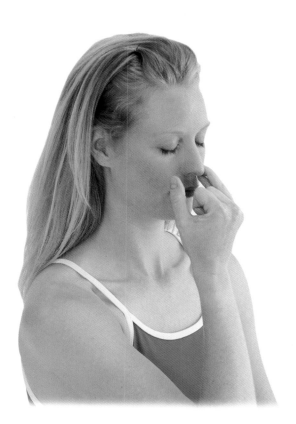

explore*yoga*

Once your Nadi Suddhi practice develops, implement a count so that the inhalations and exhalations are of equal length. Choose a number or beats that is in no way stressful to keep up. Over weeks, increase the count. It should always feel flowing and natural, never strained. Force is counterproductive in pranayama so if you find yourself tensing, then reduce the count.

Nostril Dominance

You might notice that one nostril feels more open than the other. Each nostril relates to an energy channel (nadi) which, according to esoteric anatomy, runs up the side of the vertebral column. The right nostril corresponds to the Pingala Nadi, which is more intellectually alert, aware, active; a more "masculine" energy similar to the yang of Chinese medicine. It is the perfect nostril to have open during an exam as it relates to intellectual pursuits, rational thought, attention to detail, vigorous physical action, and digesting food. The left nostril relates to the Ida Nadi and corresponds to the "feminine" (yin) traits of intuition, creative processes, holistic and imaginative thinking. It would be a good nostril to have open when you need to make a subjective decision, play music, or when you need slow, sustained energy expenditure. Nadi Suddhi pranayama helps balance these two important pranic pathways. To test which nadi is more active at any time, place the back of the hand under the nose and exhale over it.

Dominance changes at about 30- to 120-minute intervals throughout the day. Nostril dominance is affected by eating, emotions and fatigue. If you are having trouble falling asleep at night, you should check to see if the right nostril is dominant; if it is, switch to the left. To change nostril dominance, lie on the side opposite to the nostril you would like to open. During the day, a taking a vigorous walk will open the right nostril.

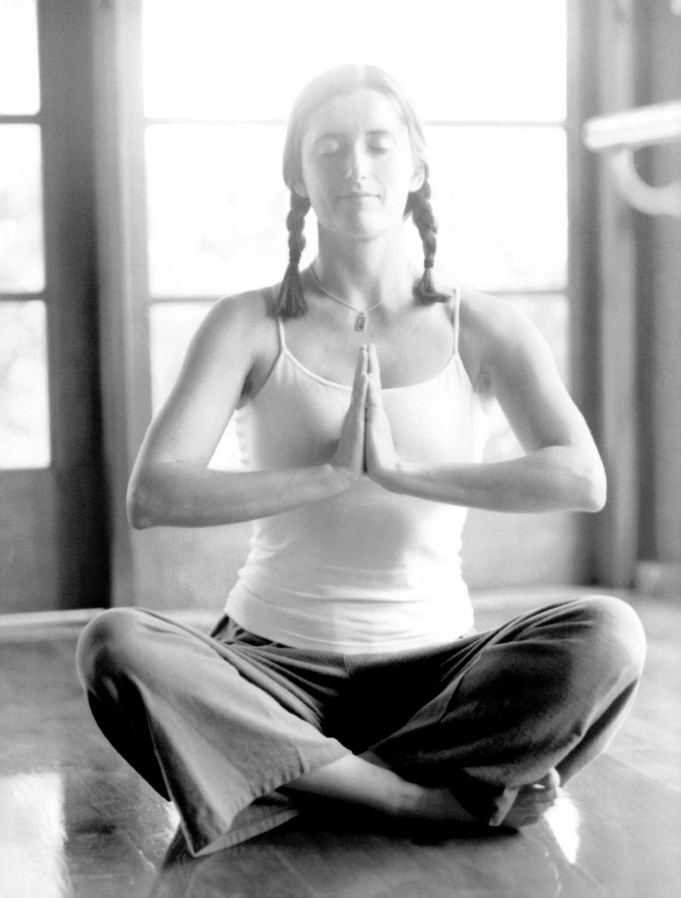

11 Meditation

On a cloudy day the sun seems like a dull light behind a haze
of white. When the sun can't be seen clearly, it's easy to forget,
or doubt, its presence. Yet, the sun never stops shining.
Meditation wipes away the cloudy veil—the false perceptions,
the illusions—and makes you receptive to the touch of pure
sunlight, the ever-present bliss state.

quieting the *mind*

Occasionally, you may find yourself with longer than 10 minutes free for meditation. While those moments are great opportunities to combine the asanas, relaxation, and breathing techniques described thus far, you will benefit greatly from setting aside some of these times for meditation, particularly if it can become a regular time.

During meditation the mind is alert and aware in a slow, effortless way. It is focused solely on one point, to contemplate and become absorbed in the formless Self. As the Self integrates into the universal spirit, meditation is expansive. It is listening instead of doing, acting, or imposing. It is observing and letting the mind be receptive to reality. Like wiping clean a dusty mirror, meditation opens you to perceive the true reflection of universal reality.

In the *Yoga-Sutras*, an early text, yoga is defined as the restraint of the chitta-vrtti—the fluctuations of the mind. In the state of yoga modifications in the thought patterns will cease. Meditation helps to still the chitta-vrtti, and attain the state of yoga.

In a meditative state, the brain wave patterns change from the beta waves of the normal awake state, to the alpha waves of deeper relaxation. Regular meditators also show theta brain waves, which occur in a state of rest deeper than sleep, but in these states, the meditator is fully aware and conscious. As the two hemispheres of the brain synchronize, mental efficiency, cognitive, and perceptual ability is increased—a study has even demonstrated meditation over a period of several years to increase the IQ.

Studies have shown impressive physiological effects of meditation. It has been shown to slow the aging process, lower blood pressure, decrease heart disease, breast cancer, osteoporosis, and reduce stress related disorders such as insomnia and depression.

Stilling the mind is not an easy task. The Vedas, the earliest known compilations of Indian spiritual writings, say the mind is harder to control than the wind. Yet long-term meditators certainly feel that meditation improves

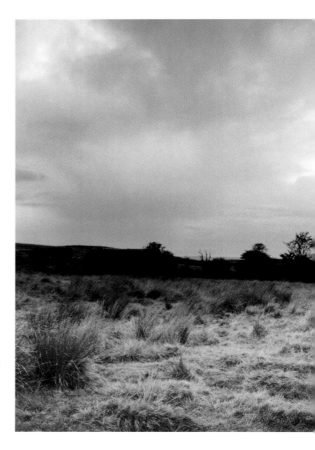

their quality of life. It brings a sense of relief and recentering, like coming home after a long and difficult journey. Self-awareness deepens and perspective is gained. In some ways, day-to-day worries are transcended. There is an inner joy that comes with this superconscious state of detaching from worldly things and developing an objective observation. Because during meditation you are aligning yourself with a positive, universal energy, something greater than yourself, meditation is a source of great inner strength.

Meditation can promote
a deep sense of inner joy.

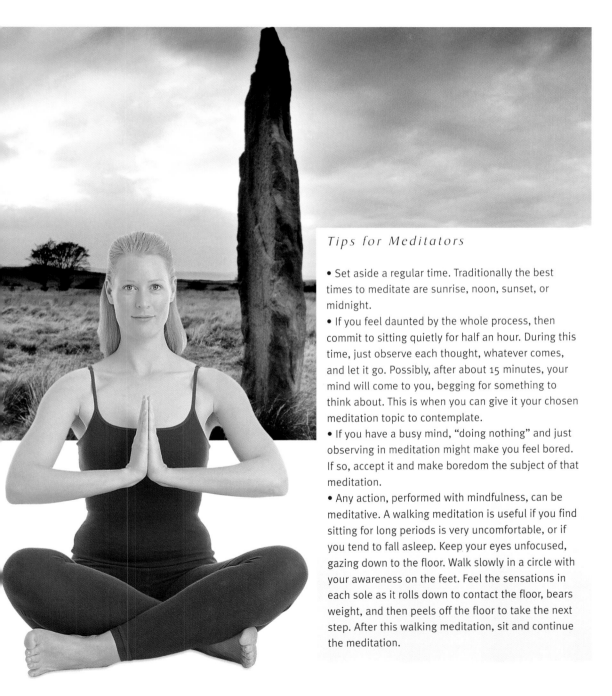

Tips for Meditators

• Set aside a regular time. Traditionally the best times to meditate are sunrise, noon, sunset, or midnight.

• If you feel daunted by the whole process, then commit to sitting quietly for half an hour. During this time, just observe each thought, whatever comes, and let it go. Possibly, after about 15 minutes, your mind will come to you, begging for something to think about. This is when you can give it your chosen meditation topic to contemplate.

• If you have a busy mind, "doing nothing" and just observing in meditation might make you feel bored. If so, accept it and make boredom the subject of that meditation.

• Any action, performed with mindfulness, can be meditative. A walking meditation is useful if you find sitting for long periods is very uncomfortable, or if you tend to fall asleep. Keep your eyes unfocused, gazing down to the floor. Walk slowly in a circle with your awareness on the feet. Feel the sensations in each sole as it rolls down to contact the floor, bears weight, and then peels off the floor to take the next step. After this walking meditation, sit and continue the meditation.

five steps for *meditation*

If you can dedicate at least 10 minutes of your day to meditation practice, in time you will be able to reap the physiological, mental, and emotional rewards.

Relax Your Body

Yoga asana practice was originally designed to let the body sit comfortably in meditation. Short of a full asana practice, do a few stretches to increase your body awareness. Take a comfortable seated position with back, neck and head erect. (See page 107 for instructions on how to sit.) If it feels right for you, offer a personal prayer, or chant to begin the session. Sweep your mind over your body, systematically relaxing each part from bottom to top. You can even do a full Savasana (see page 20) before sitting up to begin your meditation.

Once you have chosen the position that is most comfortable to you, you should avoid making any further movements since these will only act as a distraction during your meditation. When you are sitting perfectly still, every physical sensation can feel like it is intensely magnified. A small itch can become a huge torment. Breathe through these transitory sensations as they arise.

Relax Your Mind

Take three cleansing breaths by inhaling through the nose and exhaling through the mouth. Use a sigh as you exhale to release fatigue or tension. Now practise three rounds of Nadi Suddhi Pranayama (see page 114). Pay particular attention to the counting process. As with pranayama, strain is counterproductive to meditation. Keep the process relaxed.

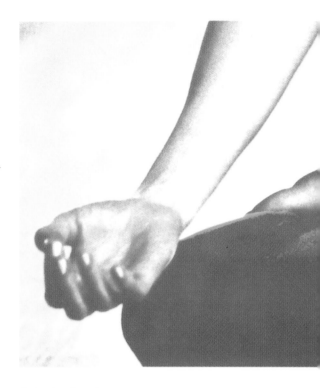

Interiorization

The breath or a mantra are useful tools to increase your concentration. You could use the ancient sound 'Om' to help focus your mind. Begin by chanting this mantra aloud, change to whispering it, then finally repeat it only in your mind.

If instead you choose to use the breath as your aid, begin by observing the flow of air through the nostrils. The cool air flows in though the nose, and the warmer air flows out. In time, follow the cool inhaled air from the nose, to the trachea. Continue to observe without any hurry. Don't alter your breath, simply be aware of what is. Possibly you can follow the flow as far down as your bronchial tubes and the lungs. On each exhalation, observe the warmed air flowing out through the nostrils from inside the body.

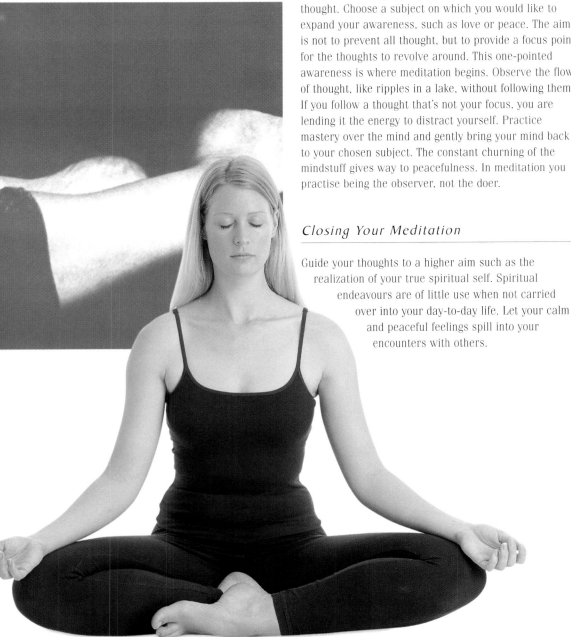

Sitting in the Lotus position is, for some, the most comfortable way to meditate.

Expand Your Consciousness

The mind has random thoughts, spreading over many subjects. The concentration in stage three confined the thoughts to a single subject—a mantra or the breath. This next step further refines it. From having many thoughts on a single subject, there is now a single thought. Choose a subject on which you would like to expand your awareness, such as love or peace. The aim is not to prevent all thought, but to provide a focus point for the thoughts to revolve around. This one-pointed awareness is where meditation begins. Observe the flow of thought, like ripples in a lake, without following them. If you follow a thought that's not your focus, you are lending it the energy to distract yourself. Practice mastery over the mind and gently bring your mind back to your chosen subject. The constant churning of the mindstuff gives way to peacefulness. In meditation you practise being the observer, not the doer.

Closing Your Meditation

Guide your thoughts to a higher aim such as the realization of your true spiritual self. Spiritual endeavours are of little use when not carried over into your day-to-day life. Let your calm and peaceful feelings spill into your encounters with others.

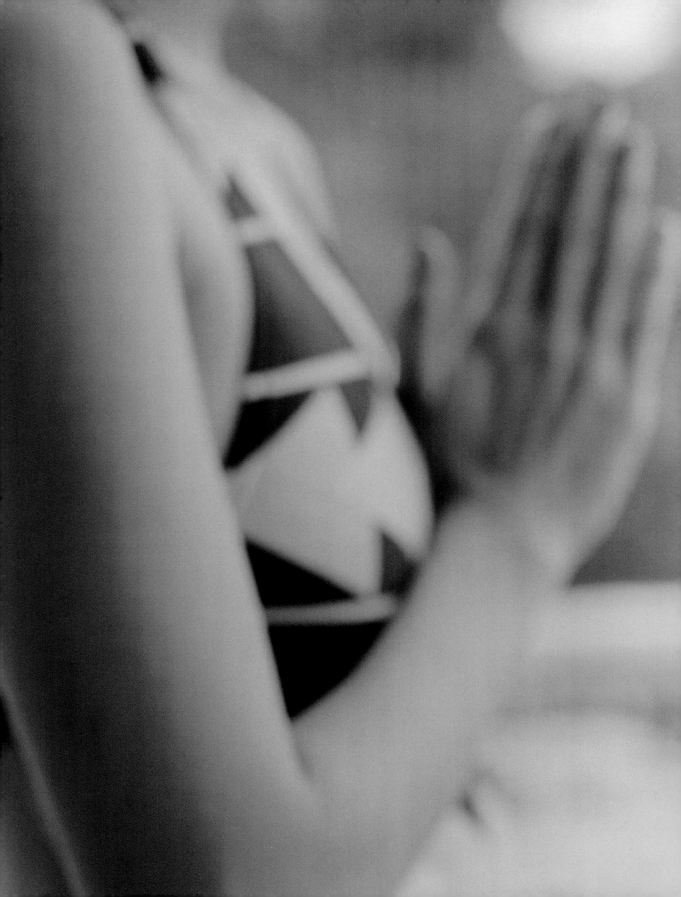

12 Therapeutic Yoga

Real health lies beyond the standard medical definition of "the absence of disease." True health encompasses a state of supreme well-being and vitality on the physical, mental, and spiritual levels.

yoga for *health*

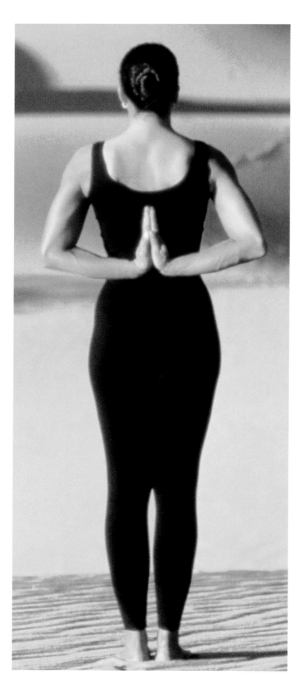

Yoga assists in the cure of diseases in a variety of ways. Each asana has specific structural and functional effects on the body. Yoga asanas promote the natural pulsations in the body. These rhythms assist circulation, increasing vitality in each cell, tissue, organ, and system.

Yoga helps to balance the hormonal and nervous systems. It balances the parasympathetic nervous system, involved in the "restore and repair" response to aid healing.

Learning deep relaxation is curative on many levels. Regular pranayama and meditation assist the mental and emotional response of the person to his or her disease.

Yoga as therapy for disease takes a holistic approach, considering each person as an individual. Indians consider each person has five koshas, or sheaths: physical, pranic, mental, intellectual, and bliss. Ill-health results from a disharmony in the koshas, which yoga helps to rebalance. Each of the following practices—cleansing techniques, postures, breath work, meditation, analysis, experience, chanting, devotion, and relaxation—promotes health through its actions on one or more of the koshas.

The table on pages 126–7 shows suggested asanas for a range of common ailments. A holistic approach aims to correct the cause of a condition and this information is intended as a guide only, not as a substitute for advice from a qualified medical practitioner.

Regular relaxation and meditation help maintain mental and physical health.

common *ailments* and *conditions*

If you suffer from one or more of the following common ailments or conditions, it is important to consider the following advice or consult a qualified health practitioner before practising yoga.

arthritis If it is difficult to hold a pose, don't stay long in it. Develop mobility in the joints by moving in and out of the pose with easy flowing movements. Avoid moving into the pain; use props if necessary.

asthma Pranayama practice will retrain the breath. Back bends are useful as they lift and open the chest, encouraging fuller breathing. Avoid caving in the chest while practicing forward bends.

anxiety Practice conscious breathing throughout the day to shift your thoughts from concerns and bring you back to the present. Physically work stress out with the asanas and perform them with as much mental focus as possible. After asanas, have a long Savasana and perform Nadi Suddhi Pranayama.

constipation Find the cause. Check your intake of fluid and dietary fiber are adequate. Sun salutation, inversions, and twists stimulate the digestive system and encourage elimination.

depression To help stay in the present moment, keep the eyes open during asana practice. Avoid forward bends as they tend to make you more introspective.

diabetes Twists and back bends tone the pancreas. Yoga asanas increase circulation and overall vitality.

fatigue Rest mental fatigue with forward bends and Savasana. Re-energize with pranayama.

herniated spinal disc Yoga can effectively manage slipped discs. Forward bending can seriously aggravate a slipped disc so hamstring flexibility needs to be developed and the back kept concave while bending forward. Support the area by strengthening the abdominal muscles.

hypertension Practice Savasana, pranayama, and meditation. But practice inversions and back bends only under the guidance of an experienced yoga teacher.

immune support After asana practice, take extra time for Savasana and pranayama. While asana practice encourages health on the cellular level, Savasana greatly assists healing on a deep level.

insomnia Both mind and body rest more easily after being extended. Do energizing asanas like Surya Namaskar and back bends in the mornings. Closer to bedtime, focus on forward bends and inversions. Take a long Savasana.

lower back strain Lower back pain has many causes and it is essential to get a correct diagnosis. While bending backward may alleviate one condition, it could aggravate another. Work with an experienced teacher to find what is appropriate.

menstrual disorders Back bends, forward bends, twists, and Surya Namaskar increase vitality to the pelvis. Inverted postures help balance hormones.

yoga during menstruation Inversions, strong twists, and strong back bends should not be practiced during menstruation. Forward bends and relaxation are recommended during this time.

yoga for the elderly Although the poses might not be as extended as those shown here, performing them with awareness will bring the same benefits. Flowing into and out of poses, rather than holding them, will develop strength. Use props if necessary, e.g. hold the wall for balance in standing postures.

obesity Sun salutation will help burn energy. Practice standing poses, back bends and inversions.

pregnancy Yoga can assist pregnancy and labor. If you are new to yoga, do not begin yoga in the first trimester. Attend a special pre-natal yoga class to learn the necessary asana modifications through the pregnancy.

stress Some mental stress can be physically worked out in the asanas. Concentrating on body awareness during asana practice gives a mental break from worrying about other things. Long Savasana releases mental and physical tension. Pranayama calms the nervous system.

therapeutic*yoga*

This chart shows which asanas are helpful for which conditions or ailments.

● Recommended
▲ Not recommended

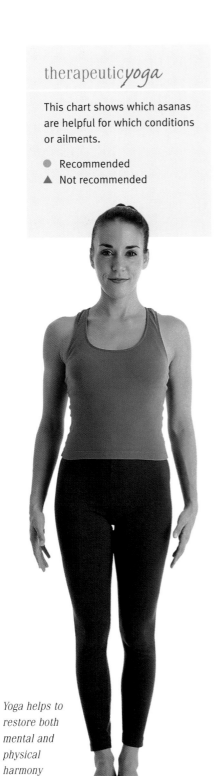

Yoga helps to restore both mental and physical harmony to the body.

	Biralasana	Awareness of breath	Standing postures	Bhujangasana	Salabhasana	Setu bandhasana
Anxiety	●	●	●	●	●	●
Arthritis	●	●	●	●	●	
Asthma	●	●		●		●
Constipation		●		●		
Depression			●	●	●	●
Diabetes		●				●
Fatigue						
Herniated spinal disc		●		●	●	●
Hypertension	●	●	▲		▲	
Immune support				●		●
Insomnia						
Lower back strain	●	●	●			
Menstrual disorders	●					●
Obesity			●	●	●	●
Pregnancy	●	●				
Stress	●	●	●	●	●	●
Yoga during menstruation	●	●				▲
Yoga for the elderly	●	●	●	●	●	●

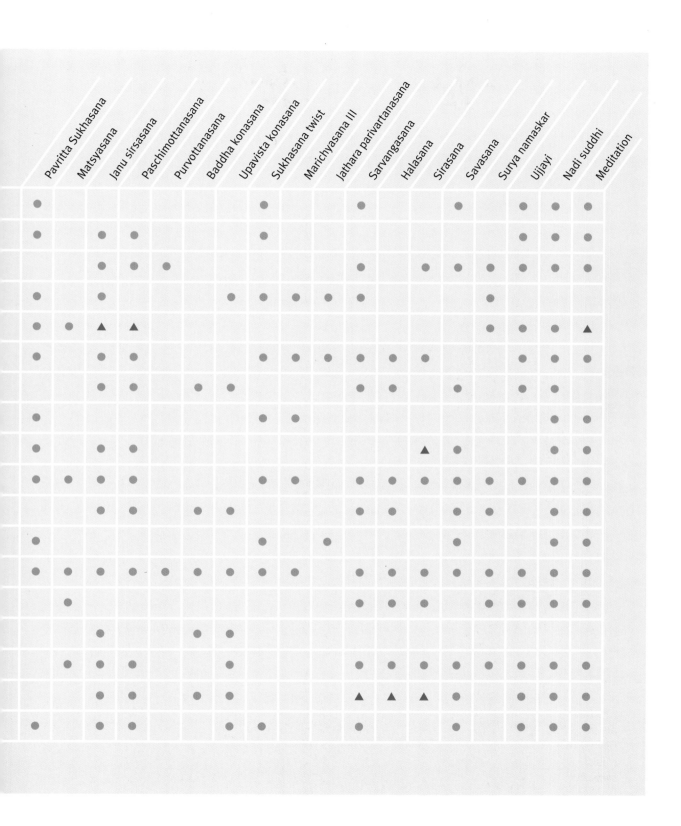

	Pavritta Sukhasana	Matsyasana	Janu sirsasana	Paschimottanasana	Purvottanasana	Baddha konasana	Upavista konasana	Sukhasana twist	Marichyasana III	Jathara parivartanasana	Sarvangasana	Halasana	Sirasana	Savasana	Surya namaskar	Ujjayi	Nadi suddhi	Meditation
	●						●				●		●		●	●	●	
	●		●	●			●									●	●	●
			●	●	●						●		●	●	●		●	
	●		●				●	●	●					●				
	●	●	▲	▲										●		●	●	▲
	●		●	●			●	●	●		●		●			●	●	●
			●	●		●	●				●		●			●	●	
	●						●	●									●	●
	●		●	●								▲	●				●	●
	●	●	●				●				●	●	●	●	●	●	●	●
			●	●			●				●	●	●	●			●	●
	●						●		●				●			●	●	●
	●	●	●	●	●	●	●	●			●	●	●	●	●	●	●	●
		●									●	●	●		●	●	●	●
			●			●	●											
		●	●	●		●	●				●	●	●	●		●	●	●
			●	●		●	●			▲	▲	▲	●			●	●	●
	●		●	●		●	●				●		●			●	●	●

index